Christian Childbirth Workbook

Christian Childbirth Workbook

By Jennifer Vanderlaan

Birthing Naturally ✢ 2010

The Christian Childbirth Workbook
© 2008 Jennifer Vanderlaan
www.birthingnaturally.net
All Rights Reserved

Published 2010 by Birthing Naturally, Colonie NY 12205
ISBN 10 0-9765541-3-5
ISBN 13 978-0-9765541-3-4

DISCLAIMER: By reading this book, you agree to educate yourself about your options and be responsible for the choices you make. The author of this book is neither a physician nor a midwife. This book has been written to help you become educated and is intended to be used in consultation with your chosen health care provider. The publisher and author accept no responsibly for any loss, damage or injury alleged to be caused by the information contained in this book. This book is not a substitute for professional prenatal care or counseling.

Dedicated to the families who have
allowing me to be a part of their birth preparation.
It has blessed me more than I could ever express.

This workbook would not have been possible without the gentle urging,
loving correction and constant encouragement of some dear old friends
and some wonderful new ones. I could never thank you ladies enough.
May this book continually bear fruit from your sacrifices.

Table of Contents

From the Author   5
How to Use this Book   7

Unit One: Stewardship   **11**
    What is eternally significant about pregnancy   12
    Changes in Mother   13
    Changes in Baby   14
    Pregnancy Exercises   15
    The Kegel Muscle   16
    Pelvic Tilt   17
    Squatting   17
    Pregnancy Nutrition   18
    Make it Nutrient Dense   19
    Quick Meal Ideas   19
    Meal Planning   20
    Stewardship of Pregnancy   21
    10 Easy Changes I Can Make   22
    Understanding My Body   23
    Productive or Unproductive   24
    More Than Meets the Eye   24
    Scripture Insight   25

Unit Two: Labor Comfort   **27**
    No Rules, No Limits   28
    Normal Labor   29
    The Experience of Labor   30
    The Labor Clock   31
    Positions for Labor   32
    Physical Comfort Measures for Labor   33
    Abdominal Breathing   34
    Spiritual Comfort Measures for Labor   35
    Love Languages in Labor   36
    Comfort Measures Assessment   37
    A Deeper Knowing   38
    God as Comforter   38
    Scripture Insight   39

Unit Three: Greeting Baby   **41**
    What is Second Stage   42
    How to Push   43
    Protect the Perineum   44
    The Immediate Post Partum   45
    Staying Comfortable While Pushing   46
    Second Stage Positions   47
    Accepting Your Adequacy   48
    Letting Go   48
    Scripture Insight   49

Unit Four: Choosing With Love — 51

- Options for Labor — 52
- Facing the Facts — 53
- Making Decisions About Interventions — 54
- Handling Medication Side Effects — 55
- Labor Story One — 56
- Labor Story Two — 57
- Discussing Options with your Caregiver — 58
- My Choices — 59
- Epidural Assessment — 60
- What Will I Choose? — 61
- Hearing the Voice of God — 62
- Making Good Use of Your Tools — 62
- Scripture Insight — 63

Unit Five: Labor Challenges — 65

- Difficult Spots in Labor — 66
- Variations of Normal Before Labor — 67
- Variations of Normal During Labor — 68
- Birth Emergencies — 68
- Handling Labor Challenges — 69
- Cesarean Surgery — 70
- Labor Challenges Role Play — 71
- Knowing the Truth — 72
- Having Peace — 72
- Scripture Insight — 73

Unit Six: Birth Planning — 75

- Writing a Birth Plan — 76
- Planning With the End in Mind — 77
- Theories of Managing Labor Pain — 78
- Fear-Tension-Pain Cycle — 79
- Cultural Beliefs — 80
- Opinions — 81
- Wise Decisions — 82
- Birth Plan Check-sheet — 83
- Setting Your Goals — 84
- God Remains in Control — 84
- Scripture Insight — 85

Unit Seven: Self-Control — 87

- Staying Comfortable — 88
- Massage Techniques to Try — 89
- Labor Rehearsal — 90
- Understanding Your Options — 91
- Labor Role Play — 92
- Self-Evaluation — 93
- Is This Labor? — 94
- God's Timing — 94
- Scripture Insight — 95

Unit Eight: Parenting a Newborn   **97**

    What the Mother May Experience Postpartum   98
    Danger Signs   98
    What Your Baby May Experience Postpartum   99
    Concerns About Your Baby   100
    What Your Newborn Needs   100
    Circumcision   101
    The Amazing Newborn   102
    Breast Feeding   103
    Postpartum Depression   104
    Support Identification   105
    Ministry of Motherhood   106
    Parenting   106
    Scripture Insight   107

From the Author

It gives me great pleasure to congratulate you on your new baby. Whether this is your first child, or you are a well-seasoned parent, the expectation of a new baby brings hearts and minds back to the center of who we are. You may find yourself asking what your purpose on Earth may be. Or you may fear you do not trust God enough. You may wonder if you are adequate as a parent, or what you will pass on to your children. Because you are using Christian materials, you may even be wondering if you are Christian "enough" to have a Christian childbirth.

I want to ease your mind because Christian childbirth is not about what positions or comfort techniques you choose. Christian childbirth is not about learning super spiritual methods to manage pain or about having a specific outcome. Christian childbirth is about growing closer to God through your childbearing experience, which is exactly what this workbook is designed to help you do.

As you learn about your body, plan for your baby's birth and study your options, you will also be challenged to reexamine what you know and assume about living a Christian life. You will question your motives and compare your heart to the heart of Christ. The one thing you will not do through this book is learn to think just like I do. This is for two reasons.

First, I have no reason to believe my inherently flawed understanding of God is any better than your inherently flawed understanding. None of us is perfect. There is always room for growth, even among the most mature Christians.

Secondly, I trust God to lead you where you need to be. You and I may struggle with the same fears, or we may have completely different struggles. You may need to hear the things God has taught me in some areas, and be five steps ahead of me in others. But the principles are sound, and God can use them to help you grow without my trying to guess what God wants you to work on next.

To give you the best opportunity to grow, I want to make sure you know you have permission to do three things.

You have permission to disagree with me, with your childbirth educator, doula, midwife, friends and any other people who are giving you information about childbirth. Take time to look up the verses. Share opposing thoughts and conclusions with the Bible backing you.

You have permission to doubt assumptions you have always accepted as true. Just because you have believed something since childhood does not make it true. Search the Bible to find the answers you seek. You may find you were always right, or you may find you have been wrong.

You have permission to wait. You do not need to have a full understanding of God's plan for childbirth today. n ten years you may find your understanding has deepened, grown and changed. This is normal.

So I invite you to relax, accept that only God can judge you, and dive into this study to see how much you can grow.

In your service,
Jennifer Vanderlaan

How to use this book

The Christian Childbirth Workbook is designed to fit around your plan for labor preparation. Use it to follow along in a traditional childbirth class, during a Christian childbirth class or study on your own. Here are some pointers to help you get the most out of these materials.

At the beginning of each unit you will find an overview and highlighted discussion points for the topics covered. You will also find a scripture checklist, suggested readings and self-study guide. Take your time to explore the listed verses, and add additional scriptures to the list as you work through the unit. The self-study guide provides ways to apply the information you are learning into your life through additional Bible reading, discussion with friends and family and personal reflection. The suggested readings are coordinated to help you use the Workbook with any Birthing Naturally materials you choose.

Within each unit, you will find a combination of activities and notes pages. Use the notes spaces to keep track of the information you think is important. Complete the activities to practice what you are learning and determine what additional information you may need.

The workbook pages have a margin for your thoughts. Use this space to record your reactions to the material you are learning. Think of it as a journal within the workbook. Express your thoughts however you feel comfortable. Use words, pictures or lists to express ideas, ask questions of God or highlight additional research you would like to do. Each unit ends with devotional thoughts, additional scripture to look up and prayer topics.

Although this workbook covers all the topics you need to plan and prepare for childbirth, this is not a complete childbirth class in a book. You will not be able to complete the workbook without additional learning materials because rather than giving answers, this book gives you questions. You must then decide when and how you will find the answers. There is no answer key in the back. The only way to check your research is with additional research. How you gather this information is up to you. Some families will choose to take a class, some will read books, some will hire a private teacher or doula, others will surf the internet. There is great flexibility to match your study to your learning style.

A Christian Childbirth Class

If you choose to participate in a Christian childbirth class designed around the workbook, your group facilitator will explain which pages to complete at home and which will be done together in class. Additional reading suggestions may be given to cover any topics not discussed at group meetings.

A Traditional Childbirth Class

If you choose to supplement a traditional childbirth class with the workbook, use the workbook to keep notes on the subjects covered each week. You should be able to get a schedule of topics from your facilitator which you can use to coordinate your personal and group learning. Use the time between classes to explore the rest of the topics in each unit.

A Small Group Study

If you are studying these materials as part of a small group, work through the units in the order they appear to allow for the natural building of knowledge by topic. It may be helpful to assign each member a topic to research, and that person would be facilitator for that day's meeting. You may also choose to study the physical information on your own, while focusing the group time on the Scripture Checklist at the beginning of each unit and the Scripture Insight at the end of each unit. Additional materials for small groups can be found on the Birthing Naturally web site, www.birthingnaturally.net.

A Personal Study

There are many benefits to working through this material with a group, but that is not always possible. If you decide studying the workbook alone is your best option, take notes in the workbook as you study through the suggested readings. Study as many additional materials as you feel you need to adequately answer the questions. Rather than jump from topic to topic, try to work from the start of the book to the end. If you are not studying the book with a class, it is recommended you also read the Christian Childbirth Handbook for the background information on the Christian aspects of each unit.

Resources

Not sure where to start finding the answers? The Christian Childbirth Handbook is the perfect companion to the Christian Childbirth Workbook. If that is not enough, the Birthing Naturally Web site answers many of the questions, and provides a directory of web sites to help you find additional information. Here are some of the best resources listed in the Natural Childbirth Directory.

Internet Resources

Childbirth Connection — www.childbirthconnection.org

Childbirth Connection provides information about the latest childbirth research for health care consumers. Many of their materials are available in pdf format for easy printing and reading off-line.

Waterbirth International — www.waterbirth.org

Waterbirth International provides information about giving birth in water. Research on waterbirth is available at the web site.

La Leche League — www.llli.org

La Leche League is an international leader in breast feeding research. The web site provides research based answers in multiple languages.

Lamaze International — www.lamaze.org

Within the new and expectant parents section of the web site, you will find research on healthy birth practices as well as videos depicting the use of these practices.

Hesperian Foundation — www.hesperian.org

Hesperian produces health training manuals for health workers in developing countries. You will find health information in many languages written for individuals with little medical background. Many of their titles are available to download at their web site.

World Health Organization — www.who.int

Using the Health Topics link, select maternal health. Within this section are a wide variety of resources and publications about care during pregnancy and birth, though many are written in medical language.

Printed Resources

The following books are quite thorough and will provide answers to your questions. However, it is important to remember these books are written to present research and many readers may find the material dry or hard to get through. Use the index to locate the information you want without getting bogged down.

Thinking Woman's Guide to a Better Birth by Henci Goer

Pregnancy, Childbirth and the Newborn by Penny Simkin, Janet Whalley, Ann Keppler, Janelle Durham and April Bolding

A Guide to Effective Care in Pregnancy and Childbirth by Murray Enkin, Marc J.N.C. Keirse, JAmes Neilson, Caroline Crowther, Lelia Duley, Ellen Hodnett and Justus Hofmeyr

The Labor Progress Handbook by Penny Simkin and Ruth Ancheta

The Birth Partner by Penny Simkin

Overview

This pregnancy is a gift from God. Right now you are growing and caring for one of God's children. You are accountable to God for how you use the resources he has given you to care for this child. You are also accountable to God for the decisions you make which affect this child while in your care. How you care for the things God has given you is stewardship.

To help you make the best decisions for the health of your child, you will need to educate yourself about how to keep both mother and baby healthy. Eating a nutritious diet is one of the best ways to maintain good health. Keeping your body active not only helps you feel more comfortable and energetic, but also prepares your body for labor.

You will also find you have options for how to handle the normal discomforts of pregnancy. Understanding the options available will help you be a good steward of this pregnancy.

Discussion Points

- ✓ How you treat your body is a matter of stewardship. Make the best use of the resources God has given you to keep yourself and your baby healthy.
- ✓ The quality of your diet will have a significant impact on your health.
- ✓ In general, whole foods served as close to their natural state as possible will be the best options for optimal health.
- ✓ American College of Obstetricians and Gynecologists (ACOG) recommends that pregnant women exercise daily, citing that exercise during pregnancy is linked to healthier pregnancies and fewer problems in labor.
- ✓ Many pregnancy discomforts can be handled by making changes in diet and exercise habits.

Self-Study

- ✑ Follow the principles of good nutrition and exercise for one week. How does your body feel different? What was difficult about this experience? What was enjoyable about this experience?
- ✑ Look through different directions God has given about eating. Adam and Eve (Genesis 2:16), Noah (Genesis 9:3) and Moses (Leviticus 11:3-4) were all given different guidelines. Explore what else the Bible has to say about food. In what ways does what you believe about God affect the way you eat?
- ✑ Keep a food journal for one to three days. Enter this information into a free online nutrition analysis program. How does your nutrition stack up?

Unit One
Stewardship

Scripture Checklist
- ❏ Matthew 25:14-30
- ❏ Luke 12:47-48
- ❏ 1 Corinthians 6:19-20
- ❏ Jeremiah 10:23
- ❏ 2 Corinthians 5:15
- ❏ Psalm 24:1
- ❏ Luke 16:10
- ❏ 1 Corinthians 4:2
- ❏ Galatians 6:9
- ❏ Matthew 6:19-20
- ❏ Psalm 193:14
- ❏
- ❏
- ❏
- ❏

Suggested Readings

Christian Childbirth Handbook
What is Christian Childbirth?
Healthy Pregnancy

40 Weeks
Part One: Healthy Pregnancy

Birthing Naturally Web site
Pregnancy Exercise
Pregnancy Nutrition

Unit One
Stewardship

My Thoughts...

What is eternally significant about pregnancy?

Matthew 6:19-20 calls us to seek out that which is eternally significant. The question is, "What exactly is eternally significant about pregnancy?"

> ⇒ STORE TREASURES IN HEAVEN
>
> SPREADING GOD'S GLORY

What are some ways you can use this time of pregnancy to:
Build your faith?

> TRUST

Give glory to God?

> THANKFULNESS

Mature spiritually?

> TRUST | RELIANCE

Witness to those around you?

> HOPE | SECURITY

This unit focuses on the eternal significance of the decisions you make. Though specific decisions may not be significant in themselves, the process you use to make the decision can reveal where your heart is. Are you making decisions as a good steward of what God has given you, or are you making decisions to serve yourself. It all comes down to stewardship. Did you do your best with what God put in your care?

Discussion Question:
Reflecting on the decisions you have already made for this pregnancy, what is revealed about your heart by the way you make decisions?

Changes in Mother

Pregnancy changes the mother's circulating levels of progesterone and estrogen which is essential to maintain a pregnancy. However, the increased progesterone levels also cause some changes in the mother's body. List some things you can do to minimize the discomforts caused by these changes.

Digestion
Your digestive system is relaxed by progesterone. This can make digestion sluggish causing heartburn and constipation.

- MORE FIBER
- EXERCISE

Circulation
Your circulatory system is also made of smooth muscle and so is relaxed by progesterone. Your body increases the amount of circulating blood during pregnancy. Your heart pumps more blood, faster than it did before you were pregnant. You may feel dizzy in extreme heat or when you stand up fast. Your body may feel puffy due to the increased circulation.

- SLOW TO STAND

Breasts
Progesterone and estrogen stimulate your mammary glands to mature and prepare to produce milk. This may cause tenderness and sensitivity as well as an increase in breast size.

- BIGGER BRA

Respiration
Progesterone also causes your lung capacity to increase to meet the increased need for oxygen and to remove carbon dioxide. You may notice you breathe faster and your rib cage has expanded.

- LOOSER CLOTHING

Unit One
Stewardship
My Thoughts...

**Unit One
Stewardship**

My Thoughts...

Changes in Baby

Your baby begins growing and forming from the moment of conception. The internal organs are formed by the 10th week of pregnancy, however most systems will continue to mature as your baby grows. Here are some highlights of your baby's development. (Weeks are given in gestational time, about two weeks behind your pregnancy week.)

Day 1: Fertilization, the sperm and egg meet and begin to make your baby.

Day 10: Your baby implants in the uterine wall.

Week 2: The bag of waters forms around your baby. The placenta begins to form and grow to bring food, water and oxygen to your baby.

Week 3: Lung buds, heart and central nervous system begin to form.

Week 4: Face and internal organs begin to develop. Circulation begins.

Week 5: External ears, eyes, nose, arm and leg buds begin to develop. Brain and spinal cord are well developed. Baby's blood vessels are working.

Week 6: Testes or Ovaries develop. Vertebrae are laid down, and there is rapid brain growth. Only 1/4 inch long.

Week 7: Nasal openings, fingers and toes, muscle fibers begin to develop.

Week 8: Human facial features well developed. Teeth form. Penis appears.

Week 9: Mini human look. Major blood vessels almost formed. Just over one inch long.

At the End of:

3 Months: Baby has primitive hair follicles and finger nails. Baby can make fists, open mouth, squint face and is about 3 inches long.

4 Months: Baby has a mini adult brain. Her eyebrows and lashes are growing. The heartbeat is audible with a stethoscope. Baby is 8 ½ inches long.

5 Months: The midpoint of your pregnancy, you have probably felt the baby move. Baby has hair on his head and is skinny at 12 inches and only 1 pound. Fat is beginning to be deposited under his skin.

6 Months: Baby's skin has a protective cover called vernix. Baby's eyes open and will soon be sensitive to light. The ears can hear. Your baby has finger and foot prints. Baby is around 14 inches long, 2 pounds.

7 Months: Taste buds have developed, and the organs are developed well enough for him to survive. 16 inches long and 3 ½ pounds.

8 Months: Her brain is growing rapidly, and so is her body. She is putting on fat and may weigh 5 pounds and be 18 inches long.

9 Months: He is putting on fat as he waits to be born, your baby is around 7 pounds and 20 inches long. He has about an inch of hair on his head and his skin is red.

Pregnancy Exercises

Pregnancy Exercise

List the reasons to exercise during pregnancy.

- MINIMIZE WEIGHT GAIN
- EASIER LABOR
- HEALTHIER BABY

Types of Exercise

List your favorite exercises from each type.

Strength
- YOGA
- BODY WEIGHT RESISTANCE

Flexibility
- STRETCHING
- YOGA

Cardiovascular
- WALKING
- HIKING

Your Exercise Schedule:

Think about your daily schedule. Are there days you have more or less time for activity? Are there ways you can adjust your schedule to increase the amount of activity? Write out a sample exercise schedule here:

Monday

Tuesday

Wednesday

Thursday

Friday

Saturday

Sunday

Unit One
Stewardship

My Thoughts...

Unit One
Stewardship

My Thoughts...

The Kegel Muscle

Label the pelvic structures.

Bladder

Cervix

Coccyx

Pelvic Floor (Kegel) Muscle

Rectum

Uterus

Vagina

Why do Kegel exercises?

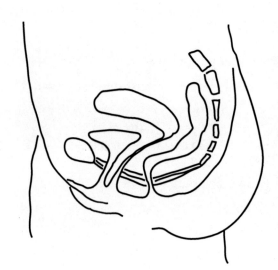

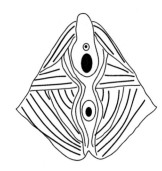

How to do it

To begin, try to isolate the pelvic floor by contracting it as if you were trying to stop the flow of urine. Do not worry at first about letting go of the contraction; just let it relax on its own. As you get stronger you will learn how to let go of the contraction.

Begin building the strength of the muscle by holding the contraction for 1 second, then 2 seconds and eventually up to 3 seconds.

When you are strong enough to hold the contraction for 3 seconds, increase your control of the muscle by contracting a little, then a little more, then all the way. Learn to contract the muscle in increments before you begin to learn to relax the muscle in increments.

The last step is to learn to relax, or bulge the muscle. This is the same movement you use to release the flow of urine. After contracting the muscle, bulge it out (if you have difficulty determining if the muscle is bulged, put your hand along the perineum. You should feel it bulge out as you relax the Kegel muscle)

Pelvic Tilt

Why Pelvic Tilt?

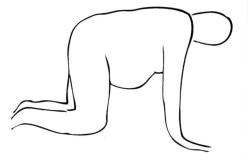

How to do it

While on hands and knees, tilt your pelvis under by contracting deep abdominal muscles. While you are learning, try to pay close attention to the abdominal contraction. This will prevent you from trying to tilt your pelvis by arching your back. When it is done properly, the movement is very small and your back should stay relatively flat.

Squatting

Why Squat?

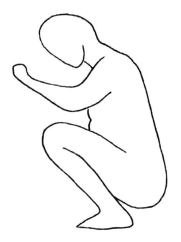

How to do it

Keeping your feet firmly planted on the floor, lower your upper body into a slight bend; lower your bottom to the floor by bending your knees and hips.

If you find it is difficult to keep your balance, stand in front of a table, counter, heavy chair or another person, and hold on while you lower your body.

Unit One
Stewardship

My Thoughts...

Pregnancy Nutrition

Various Recommendations for Adequate Nutrition in Pregnancy

Food Group	Dr. Brewer	USA	Canada	Australia	UK
Protein	4	2-3	2	1.5	Moderate
Dairy	4	2	2	2	2-3
Fruits and Vegetables	5	5-9	7-8	9-10	5
Grains	4	6-11	6-7	4-6	1/3 of diet
Pregnancy Specific	NA	1 additional dairy serving	Add 2-3 servings of any group	NA	NA

Why do you need each type of nutrient?

Protein:

Carbohydrates:

Fat:

Discussion Questions:
What concerns do you have about the way you eat?
What drives your decisions about what to eat?

Make it Nutrient Dense

What can you add to make these foods more nutrient dense? List your favorite food additions for each category.

Add to Salads:

Add to Sandwiches:

Add to Soups:

Add to Baked Goods:

List your favorite nutrient dense snacks.

List your favorite nutrient dense side dishes.

List your favorite nutrient dense toppings.

Quick Meal Ideas

Which of these quick meal ideas fit into your lifestyle?
- Bowl of Cereal, toast with peanut butter, glass of milk
- Cottage cheese with fruit
- Yogurt with fruit and granola
- Grilled cheese sandwich, salad or fresh vegetables
- Slice of cheese, English muffin or toast, piece of fruit
- Tuna sandwich, fruit
- Mixed nuts, piece of cheese, glass of juice
- Dry cereal with yogurt
- Peanut Butter and Jelly sandwich, fresh vegetables
- Instant soup or can of soup
- Popcorn, piece of cheese, piece of fruit

Add more ideas:

Unit One
Stewardship
My Thoughts...

Unit One
Stewardship

My Thoughts...

Meal Planning

Plan three days of meals following the dietary recommendations.

	Day One	Day Two	Day Three
Breakfast			
Morning Snack			
Lunch			
Afternoon Snack			
Dinner			
Evening Snack			

Pointers:

Think outside the dinner plate. Six smaller meals may work better for you than 3 large meals.

Use the foods you know you like. You do not have to eat chicken if you hate it.

Double a recipe and use the leftovers for a lunch or freeze them for a quick dinner later in the month.

Eggs are not just a breakfast food. Keep deviled or hard boiled eggs for quick snacks.

Discussion Question:
How easy or difficult was it to create a nutritious menu?

My Thoughts...

Stewardship of Pregnancy

Your pregnancy and your baby will change your life in many ways. Some changes you may have expected, others may have come as a surprise to you. Take a few minutes to consider ways your life has changed since becoming pregnant, and the ways it will change after your baby is born. List the changes in the appropriate area of the diagram below. Consider how these changes affect your other responsibilities, and what you can do to prepare for them.

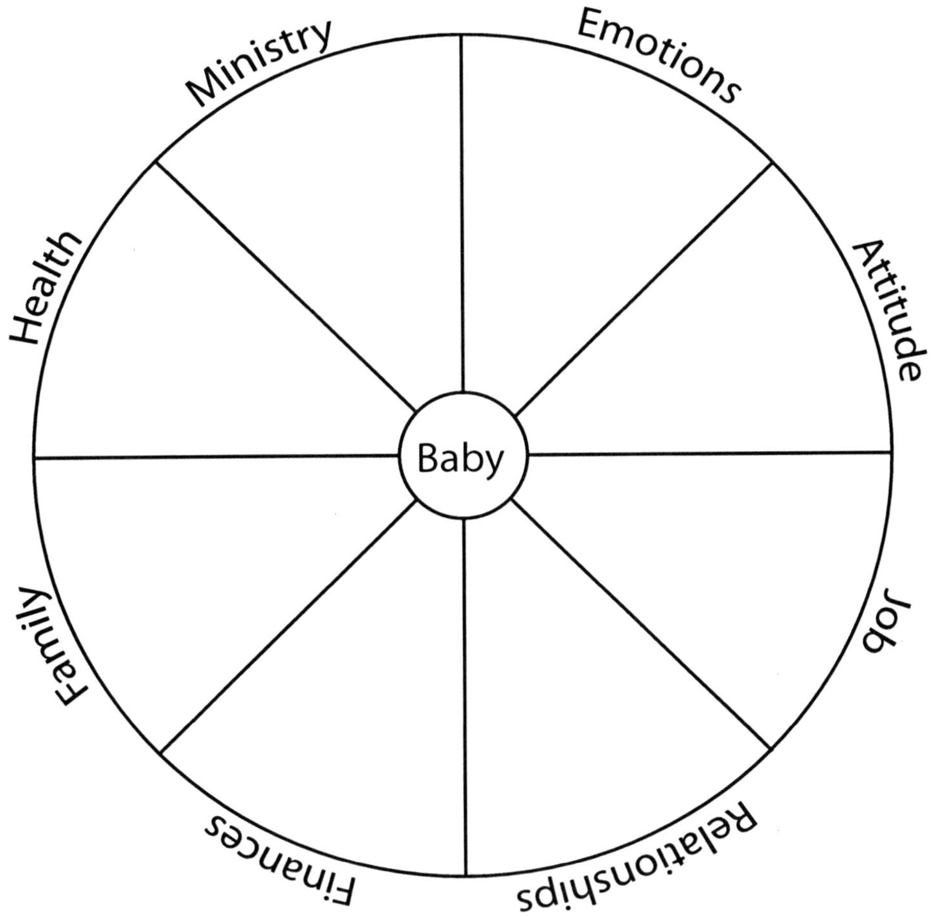
Ministry
Emotions
Attitude
Job
Relationships
Finances
Family
Health
Baby

Discussion Question:
What possible changes have you anticipated?
How can you be prepared for those changes?

Unit One
Stewardship

My Thoughts...

10 Easy Changes I Can Make

Please list 10 specific things you can do in your everyday life to improve your health during this pregnancy. Instead of saying "eat healthy," say what you will do such as keep cut vegetables in the refrigerator.

1.

2.

3.

4.

5.

6.

7.

8.

9.

10.

Understanding My Body

This worksheet is designed to help you prepare for the upcoming birth by identifying the way your body handles stress and pain. You should think about all sources of stress or discomfort, physical and emotional. Think of recent situations you have been in and consider how you responded to those situations.

I know I am feeling tense or stressed when my body…

My body reacts to tension by…

To remain clam while stressed I…

To cope with pain, I prefer…

Be Alone	or	Be With People
Keep Myself Busy	or	Tune Into Myself
Distract My Thoughts	or	Explore My Thoughts
Be Quiet	or	Talk With Someone
To be Touched	or	Not to Be Touched
Have Someone Help	or	Work it Out Alone

What has been your experience with using the following stress and pain coping techniques?

- Slow Deep Breathing

- Massage

- Visualization or Meditation on Scripture

- Vocalization

- Progressive Relaxation

- Using a Focus Point

- Prayer

Unit One
Stewardship
My Thoughts…

Circle your stress responses:

Head
Tension Headache
Tired Eyes
Grinding Teeth
Clenching Jaw
Ringing in Ears

Neck
Muscle Tightness
Decreased Range of Motion

Shoulders/Arms
Muscle Tightness
Trembling Hands
Gripping Fists
Biting Nails

Chest
Heart rate increasing
Heart pounding
Difficulty catching breath

Stomach
"Butterflies" in Stomach
Nausea

Back
Muscle Tightness
Sore Back
Bad Posture

Skin
Sweating
Clammy Skin
Itching/Scratching

Legs/Feet
Bouncing Legs
Trembling Feet
Sore or Achy Feet
Muscle Tension

Mental Processes
Speech Difficulties
Inability to Focus

Unit One
Stewardship
My Thoughts...

Productive or Unproductive

A healthy concern can be productive, encouraging you to make the healthiest decisions for yourself and your baby. Such concern is a motivator, moving us to do the things God desires for us to do.

Learning how to handle the challenges of labor is what drives most women to childbirth classes. Labor and birth have become so separate from our lives that very few women have actually seen a birth before their first child is born. Because of this, a normal healthy concern to be as prepared as possible can be helpful.

Yet for some women, concern becomes an unproductive fear, paralyzing them from making decisions or enjoying the blessings of a pregnancy. In addition to preventing proper preparation, such fears can cause problems during a labor. The female body is designed to stop labor in unsafe situations. Regardless of the cause, fear is a trigger for stopping labor.

There are a lot of unknowns in labor because you are not in control. Yet you can take comfort in knowing God is in control. Even if the task set before you is difficult, God will give you the strength to come through it.

Do not confuse a lack of concern with trusting God. Judge how much you are trusting God by looking at every area of your life, not just pregnancy. It is possible to feel a lack of concern because you are choosing to avoid the reality of the situation. Avoidance may be another form of fear.

In short, your faith in God is not exhibited by the lack of concern for labor, but in your continuing to act according to the will of God regardless of what is going on around you.

More Than Meets the Eye

You are more than just a bag of flesh. You are a body and spirit, and both parts of you will be challenged during labor. You will learn to master physical comfort techniques with a little practice. It will take much more than practice to master spiritual comfort.

Spiritual comfort comes from peace and trust, perseverance and resting in the Lord. These are more than simple attitudes to adopt during labor; they are the evidence of a heart that loves and serves God alone.

Your spiritual comfort must be built before labor begins. It comes from spending time with God through Bible reading and prayer. It comes from confessing any sins you may have hidden in your heart, being honest about fears and thanking God for who he is and what he has done. Spiritual comfort comes from recognizing the true power and nature of God, and finding rest in him alone.

Spiritual comfort will not come from doing the "right things" in labor; it only exists where the heart is truly serving God.

Scripture Insight

Read Genesis 2-4, answering these questions.

1. When did God create human reproduction?

2. When then, were menstruation, pregnancy and child birth designed?

3. What or who did God curse?

4. What were the consequences for the man?

5. What were the consequences for the woman?

6. Compare the general impressions of the work of gardening to the work of giving birth.

7. What was Eve's response to the birth of a child?

To Pray About

How has your life demonstrated good stewardship, either during this pregnancy or before?

What unique opportunities for stewardship have arisen during this pregnancy?

What areas are the most difficult for you to practice good stewardship?

Unit One
Stewardship

My Thoughts...

Peace and Strength

Psalm 119:165

Isaiah 30:15

John 14:27

Philippians 4:6-7

Philippians 4:13

2 Timothy 1:7

Unit Two
Labor Comfort

Scripture Checklist
- ☐ Isaiah 30:15
- ☐ Psalm 119:165
- ☐ John 14:27
- ☐ Philippians 4:6-8
- ☐ Isaiah 26:3
- ☐ 2 Timothy 1:7
- ☐ Philippians 4:13
- ☐ Ecclesiastes 3:1-8
- ☐
- ☐
- ☐
- ☐

Overview

This unit focuses on learning how to manage labor in comfort and peace. The process of labor and what you can do to stay as comfortable as possible during labor are important things to understand. To effectively use any of these comfort measures in labor, you will need to practice them enough that you can do them while in pain and in a distracting environment.

Spiritual comfort does not come from practicing tricks and techniques to use when life is not going your way. Peace cannot be practiced or taught. True peace comes from a heart in a right relationship with God. For this reason your spiritual preparation for labor can and does influence your comfort during labor.

Discussion Points

- ✓ Understanding the normal process of labor can help you determine what types of physical comfort measures to use at different times in labor.
- ✓ Taking the time to discover the uniqueness of your body can help you understand what comfort measures will be most effective for you during labor.
- ✓ It may be possible that maintaining a quiet and undisturbed atmosphere could help you labor. It may also be possible that maintaining the right attitude can help you labor.
- ✓ Do not misinterpret the source of the power. The environment does not determine the spirit; it is the Spirit that determines the environment. You can have peace in the midst of a storm.
- ✓ Deep abdominal breathing (the breath of life) provides your body with the oxygen it needs to labor while it also works to keep your spirit at peace.

Self-Study

- ☙ Make a list of your most painful experiences. For each experience, write out the types of comfort measures you tried and how well they worked. What does this teach you about your body, and your needs for comfort?
- ☙ Do a topical study on God as your comforter. In what ways does God provide comfort for his people?
- ☙ Ask friends and family about the comfort measures they used in labor. How did they prepare to use them? How effective were they? What can you learn from their experiences?

Suggested Readings

Lord of Birth

Why is Labor so Bad?
Inviting God to Your Baby's Birth

Christian Childbirth Handbook

God's Design for Childbirth
Childbirth Pain
Staying Comfortable

Birthing Naturally Web site

Comfort Techniques
Labor Progress

Unit Two
Labor Comfort

My Thoughts...

No Rules, No Limits

Use this space to write, draw, outline or otherwise record your ideal birth. There are no restrictions on where you are, who is with you or what you can do. Simply think about what, in your mind, would be the perfect way for your baby to be born into your family.

Normal Labor

What does each of the following indicators reveal about the labor process? What are the generally accepted averages during normal labor?

Contractions

Calculate the frequency and duration of these contractions. Predict the next few contractions if the pattern continues.

Begins	Ends	Frequency	Duration
8:45:20	8:46:20		
8:47:19	8:48:20		
8:49:17	8:50:20		

Dilation

Effacement

Station

Cervical Position

Sketch a cervix at different stages of labor. How does the cervix change as labor progresses?

Unit Two
Labor Comfort

My Thoughts...

Unit Two
Labor Comfort

My Thoughts...

The Experience of Labor

Each stage of labor has specific physical and emotional characteristics that define it. By understanding how to interpret the signs of progress, you will be better able to make decisions about how to handle your labor. Also, each stage of labor has different challenges. Knowing ways to manage your comfort level can help you give birth with the least intervention possible.

Identify the characteristics and challenges of each stage of labor.

Pre-Labor

Early First Stage

Late First Stage

Transition

The Labor Clock

If the average labor is 12 hours, you can graphically represent an average labor on a standard clock face. In this exercise you will graph one normal labor. There is no right or wrong here. Normal lengths of labor stages are highly variable.

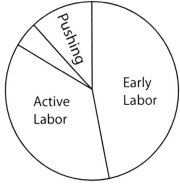

Using the circle, the line at 12:00 will be the point the baby is born. Now count backwards. What is an average pushing time? Draw a line from the center to the point on the clock that makes that time (see example). How long is an average transition? How long might a normal active labor be?

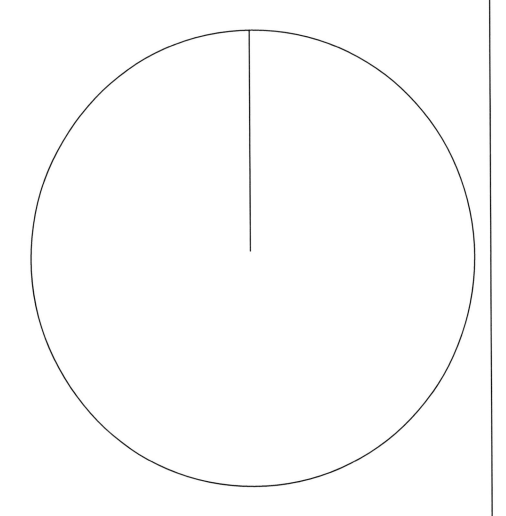

Discussion Question:
What might help you stay comfortable during each stage of labor?

Unit Two
Labor Comfort
My Thoughts...

**Unit Two
Labor Comfort**

My Thoughts...

Positions for Labor

Try each of these positions. Record your thoughts on page 37.

Upright Positions allow gravity to increase the intensity of the contractions naturally, while minimizing the discomfort.

Standing

Walking

Leaning against a wall

Dangling in someone's arms

Slow dancing

Leaning over a chair

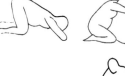

Kneeling Positions take pressure off your pelvic floor and allow the baby to change positions.

Over a chair

Over a birth ball

Into someone's lap

Over the side of a tub

Over the side of the bed

Over the end of the bed

Sitting Positions allow your body to work with gravity while allowing you to rest.

Chair, forward or backward

Beanbag Chair

Birth Ball

Floor, tailor style

Toilet

Rocking chair

Positions that give you the freedom to move your pelvis may help your baby to rotate, allowing for a faster labor.

- Try pelvic rocking in any of the upright or kneeling positions.
- Try slow dancing with a partner for support
- Sway your hips back and forth during contractions
- Try lunging forward with your foot on a chair or stool
- Try walking in between or during contractions
- Rock your hips in a figure eight during contractions
- Rock your torso back and forth as you sit

Unit Two
Labor Comfort

My Thoughts...

Physical Comfort Measures for Labor

There are many types of pain and discomfort women may feel during labor. For those not wishing to use pain relieving medications, or those waiting for the medication to take effect, the following methods of pain relief may be useful.

Try each of these comfort measures. Record your thoughts on page 37.

Heat / Cold can be applied to the area experiencing pain. The result is a dulling sensation of the pain.

Massage techniques can be used to relieve a sore back or any aching muscle.

Showers can be used to help you relax. If the stream of water is placed over the uncomfortable part of the body, the pain may lessen.

Baths can alleviate discomforts on many parts of the body at one time by relieving the weight of your body, providing heat to the areas experiencing discomfort and promoting relaxation.

Patterned Breathing can distract you from the discomfort you feel, and bring your attention away from the contraction.

Vocalization in the form of moaning, sighing, counting, singing, chanting or praying may help you relax while distracting you from your contractions. Many women find matching the volume of the vocalization to the intensity of the contraction helps them remain in control.

Abdominal Breathing helps promote relaxation and provides the body with more oxygen than chest breathing. This helps prevent fatigue and allows the muscles to work at their best.

Sleep between contractions or during early labor helps increase your stamina. You will not sleep through the birth, so sleep if you are able.

Using the Bathroom can relieve pelvic pressure by keeping the bowel and bladder empty. As the cervix dilates, you may not be able to discern if the pressure is from the cervix or a full bladder. Keeping the bladder empty can prevent some pain.

Drinking and Eating prevent dehydration and fatigue, both of which can make the contractions seem more intense and painful.

Unit Two
Labor Comfort

My Thoughts...

Abdominal Breathing

Not only does abdominal breathing enhance relaxation, it also increases the lung capacity. This means there is more oxygen for you and your baby. Abdominal breathing also uses less of your energy.

To learn to breathe abdominally, do this:

> Breathe in deeply, if your shoulders rise, you are chest breathing not abdominal breathing.

> Breathe in deeply again, this time try to push your abdominal muscles out as you breathe in.

> As you exhale, your abdominal muscles should pull back in.

How does abdominal breathing feel different from the way you normally breathe?

Spend a few minutes meditating on these scripture verses.
How does God use them to speak to you?

Job 12:10

Job 33:4

John 20:21-22

When to use Abdominal Breathing

You should use abdominal breathing throughout most of your labor. However, you may find it most useful when you:

- Feel "out of control"
- Have become frightened or stressed
- Are having difficulties relaxing
- Have lost your "focus"

Unit Two
Labor Comfort

Spiritual Comfort Measures for Labor

Comfort in labor is affected by where your mind and your spirit are focused. If you are fearful, anxious or lacking trust in God, your labor may be hindered. Unlike the physical comfort measures, spiritual comfort measures cannot be "mastered" and used during labor. Peace, confidence and faith take time to build, but once established will benefit you in every part of your life.

When you are in labor, there are ways to draw on your faith and peace of God to help you stay relaxed and confident. Just as you have a unique physical makeup, you also have a unique spiritual makeup. Some of these activities will comfort you more than others, so be sure to spend time trying each activity to see which ones help you the most. Read Isaiah 30:15, then try each of these activities. Record your thoughts on page 37.

Prayer is always good for the soul, and in labor it can be good for the body as well. Praying out loud can be used as a vocalization to match the intensity of contractions. Listening to others praying for you can give you a focus point. Pray using one of the many names used for God in the Bible; your comforter, your strength, your deliverer.

Scripture Reading gives us the chance to hear the words of God. These words can bring strength, comfort and peace. Scripture can be used as a focal point if someone else reads to you or if you read favorite verses from index cards. Reciting the verses aloud can be used as a form of vocalization, or as a distraction technique if you repeat a verse someone else reads.

Meditation can help prevent distraction, allowing you to achieve a deeper relaxation. Meditation can also be done as a form of prayer during labor. God calls us to meditate on his word, and in labor you might find it helpful to meditate on the miracle happening in your body.

Praise and Worship can help you stay focused on God. Music helps to establish a mood and is allowed at most birthing places.

Confession helps to keep us in a right relationship with God. Our sins have a disastrous effect on our relationship with God. Usually, we begin to feel guilt as a consequence of our sin. This guilt encourages us to return to the Lord. But when left unconfessed, that guilt can cause us to "hide" from God just like Adam and Eve in the garden.

My Thoughts...

Unit Two
Labor Comfort

My Thoughts...

Love Languages in Labor

Few women go into labor realizing the strongest comfort measure is the love and encouragement of those supporting her.

Dr. Gary Chapman has given us a tool to understand each other with his Five Love Languages. Dr. Chapman suggests everyone has a way in which they give and receive love most powerfully. He calls it their love language. Knowing your spouse's love language allows you to focus your efforts at showing love into those areas, which communicate love to him or her most effectively. This principle holds true even through the rigors of labor.

Which of these love languages sounds most like yours?

Quality Time:
Some women feel loved when their companions choose to be with them rather than participating in another activity. For this woman, the simple act of shutting off the television so you can talk with her speaks volumes about how valuable she is to you. To love this woman in labor, you must prevent yourself from becoming distracted and preoccupied by work, telephones, hospital procedures or other concerns.

Words of Affirmation:
Every woman needs to be told how great she is doing, but for a woman whose love language is words of affirmation, your silence during labor tells her she is alone. To love this woman in labor, you must remind her after every contraction how much you love her, how strong she is, how great she is handling labor, or how much you appreciate what she is doing.

Gifts:
For some women, the fact that someone took the time to make or purchase something for them fills their heart with joy. Although you cannot run out to purchase gifts during the labor, you can prepare ahead of time. Putting together a small photo album, a collection of poems, or a CD with favorite songs, lets this woman feel how important her laboring is to you.

Acts of Service:
When a laboring woman has the acts of service love language, everything you do to help her shows how much you care. To love her in labor, you cannot allow yourself to sit at her side while the nurses do everything. You must offer her sips of water or ice, retrieve cool or warm cloths for her face, neck and back, and be her shoulder to lean on when contractions overwhelm her.

Physical Touch:
Although most women find massage of some sort comforting in labor, some women need to be touched. For these women a back rub is an expression of your love and devotion. If she gets to the point that touching her body is no longer comfortable, you can just hold her hand.

In labor, a variety of comfort measures and pain coping techniques may need to be tried. Understanding your love language allows those with you in labor to focus their efforts on the techniques that not only keep you comfortable, but also demonstrate their love to you.

Discussion:
Can you predict helpful comfort measures based on your love language?

Unit Two
Labor Comfort

My Thoughts...

Comfort Measures Assessment

You have been working on learning a wide variety of comfort measures for labor. Because every woman is different, your response to the various techniques will be unique. Completing this assessment will help you determine which strategies are most likely to be beneficial during labor.

Technique	Comfort and confidence in my ability to do this			Success at managing pain and discomfort		
	Low	Med	High	Low	Med	High
Abdominal Breathing						
Progressive Relaxation						
Massage						
Meditation						
Visualization						
Vocalization						
Standing or Walking						
Slow Dancing						
Leaning Forward						
Sitting on Birth Ball						
Reading						
Dangling						
Effleurage						
Hip Squeeze						
Reclining or lying						
Kneeling or hands-knees						
Patterned breathing						
Counter pressure						
Hot or cold packs						
Warm shower						
Warm bath						
Talking with someone						
Distraction						
Receiving encouragement						
Physical Touch						
Music						
Prayer						
Scripture Reading						
Meditation						
Praise / Worship						

Unit Two
Labor Comfort

My Thoughts...

A Deeper Knowing

Understanding the normal process of labor can help you determine what types of comfort measures are effective at different times during labor. There are some techniques useful for speeding labor, others useful for a backache in labor and still others that can be helpful when you feel tense.

Knowing the variety of comfort measures is only the first step. Taking the time to discover the uniqueness of your body can help you understand what comfort measures are most useful for you.

Both showers and baths can have beneficial effects in labor. They can both help ease a sore back, encourage relaxation and make you more comfortable. Yet, you probably enjoy one better than the other—and knowing which you prefer is part of the key to a deeper understanding of comfort measures.

If you are a woman who finds comfort in talking about what is happening, you may choose to talk longer into your labor than most other women.

If you are a woman who prefers silence, you may choose not to use music during labor.

If you are a woman who tenses when her feet are touched, you may want to identify other parts of your body to be massaged during labor.

If you are a woman who is constantly moving, positions that limit your mobility may be less helpful for you during labor.

It all comes down to knowing who you are. Do not expect something to work for you because it worked for someone else. God created you uniquely, and it is only you who knows what really works to help you feel comfortable.

Once you have explored the different comfort measures, you will be able to share with your labor partners what are the most effective techniques for you.

God as Comforter

We have a wonderful model of a comforter in God. As early as the story of Adam (Genesis 2:20-22), we see a God who is concerned about meeting the needs of his people. God responds to Adam's lack of a companion by making Eve.

Further into the book of Genesis, we see God comforting a forlorn Hagar by meeting both her physical needs and her emotional needs (Genesis 21:17-19). He provides water for her to drink and reassurance that Ishmael will become a strong nation.

God sends comfort to Elijah by providing food and rest. After Elijah's physical needs have been met, God meets his emotional needs by reassuring him he is not alone (1 Kings 19).

It is wonderful to know God cares about our comfort. It is important to remember God seeks to meet our physical and emotional needs. As you practice comfort measures, be sure to learn techniques to bring physical and emotional comfort. Do not underestimate the importance of the emotional comfort you feel knowing God is your strength even during labor.

Scripture Insight

Read Romans 12:3-8.

1. What does it mean to be holistic?

2. What is the value of a holistic view of the body of Christ?

3. What is the value of a holistic view of the human body?

4. Explain the dangers of understanding labor as solely a work of the uterus.

5. How do other parts of the body cooperate to accomplish birth?

6. Describe the ways a labor support team works together as a body.

To Pray About

What do you need to feel comfort?
What prevents you from feeling comfortable?
How has God been your comforter?
What areas are you in need of comfort today?

Unit Two
Labor Comfort

My Thoughts...

Strength and Confidence

Psalm 51:10-12

Psalm 73:26

Psalm 119:50

Isaiah 26:3

2 Corinthians 3:4

Unit Three
Greeting Baby

Scripture Checklist
- ☐ Isaiah 57:15
- ☐ Isaiah 66:9
- ☐ Psalm 51:16-17
- ☐ Proverbs 11:2
- ☐ James 3:13
- ☐ Matthew 23:12
- ☐
- ☐
- ☐
- ☐

Overview

The process of pushing happens slowly as you work in response to your body's urges to push. During this time you must maintain a humble attitude, willing to let yourself be directed by the cues of your body. Think of it as a metaphor for following the direction of the Holy Spirit; when the Spirit says move, you move!

But just as in the rest of life, you cannot control the response your baby will have to your pushing. Your baby may come out quickly, or he may take more time as he molds and twists through the pelvis. Sometimes babies are in positions that prevent pushing from being effective. In this case, the mother will need to adjust herself to help her baby move into a better position. Once again, you will not be able to force your baby to change position, but will instead attempt to provide him an environment that allows him to change.

Here again we have a metaphor, this time for making an impact on someone else's life. Others are not always ready to change, and we must have the patience and humility to continue to love them unconditionally in the hope they will move into a position that makes them more willing to receive the truth.

Discussion Points

- ✓ The process of pushing happens slowly so the baby can mold to the pelvis. Your baby will move forward during a contraction and slip back a little between contractions.
- ✓ Certain positions your baby may assume will cause the pushing process to take longer than average.
- ✓ You cannot rush the process of pushing without increasing the risks to mother or baby. However, under some circumstances the risks of allowing the birth to happen at a slow pace are higher than the risks of rushing the process.
- ✓ Push in any position that is comfortable. Some positions may help pushing happen faster, others may help slow pushing down.

Self-Study

- ☙ Spend some time reading birth stories from the Bible. Look up the stories of Eve (Genesis 3), Hannah (1 Samuel 1), Elizabeth and Mary (Luke 1-2), Leah and Rachel (Genesis 29:31-30:24). What information can you find about the attitude of new mothers and those around them,
- ☙ Find out about the birth options in your area. Do you have hospitals, birth centers, access to homebirth? Can you hire a midwife, obstetrician or family doctor?
- ☙ Ask friends or family to share their feelings as they saw their baby for the first time. Did they experience joy or relief? Were they drawn to one feature such as eyes or hands? Did they spend hours taking pictures or talking to their new baby?

Suggested Readings
Christian Childbirth Handbook
Second Stage
Third Stage

Birthing Naturally Web site
Comfort Techniques
Labor Progress

**Unit Three
Greeting Baby
My Thoughts...**

What is second Stage?

The cervix is opened and the baby drops into the birth canal. What is important to understand about each of these parts of second stage?

Ferguson Reflex

Fetal Ejection Reflex

Pelvis

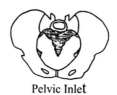 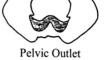

Pelvic Inlet   Pelvic Outlet

Cardinal Movements

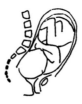 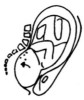 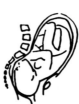 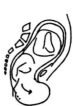 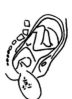

Crowning

How to Push

For some women, the fear of knowing when or how to push is the biggest fear of labor. For other women, the images of births in movies and TV have given them a faulty understanding of what the pushing process actually entails.

Reflexive Pushing

When a mother is left alone to follow her body, pushing is reflexive. Usually performed with many short pushes lasting no longer than 6 seconds each. If the contraction is stronger, the mother naturally pushes harder.

Directed Pushing

When a mother is faced with the need to give birth quickly, she is directed to take a cleansing breath, inhale deeply and push as hard as she can to the count of 10. When she reaches 10, she takes a quick breath and pushes to the count of 10 again. This gives about three long, strong pushes during a contraction.

What are the differences between these two pushing methods?
Benefits and risks:

Length of pushing time:

Breathing and vocalization:

Role of the Partner:

What is the same regardless of the pushing method used?
Use of pelvic floor muscles:

Where push is directed:

Relaxing between pushing contractions:

Discussion Question:

Read Isaiah 66:9. The idea of pushing brings fear to the hearts of many women. Why do you think women are not aware of the amazing ability of their body to stretch?

Unit Three
Greeting Baby
My Thoughts...

Unit Three
Greeting Baby

My Thoughts...

Protect the Perineum

The goal is to end labor with your skin as intact as possible, so prevention should be the focus. List ways to help keep the perineal skin intact.

Before labor begins

During labor

Do you know the arguments for natural tearing of the perineum? Do you know the arguments for episiotomy? What does the research support?

Tearing

Episiotomy

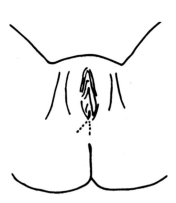

Research

The Immediate Post Partum

Things happen quickly once your baby is born. What is important to understand about each of these events?

Hormonal Changes

Breast feeding and Bonding

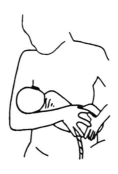

Cord Cutting

Birth of the Placenta

Repair of the Perineum

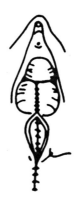

Unit Three
Greeting Baby

My Thoughts...

Unit Three
Greeting Baby

My Thoughts...

Staying Comfortable While Pushing

What does each of these have to do with staying comfortable while pushing?

Breathing and Breath Holding

Positioning

Fighting Fatigue

Lighting

Temperature (room and body)

Companions

Crowning

Second Stage Positions

Almost any position that is comfortable for the mother will work for pushing. However, there are benefits to using each type of position.

List potential benefits for each position.

Squatting Positions

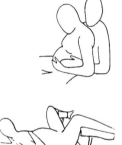

Reclining Positions

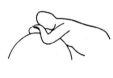

Kneeling Positions

Standing Positions

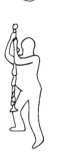

Unit Three
Greeting Baby
My Thoughts...

Unit Three
Greeting Baby

My Thoughts...

Accepting Your Adequacy

You have been created uniquely by God for the specific purposes to which he has called you. You have a unique collection of gifts, strengths, likes and abilities. You have been created for the work God determined for you before you were born. When you became a Christian, the Holy Spirit also bestowed upon you gifts for you to use in accomplishing the purposes God has for you.

Just as you have been uniquely created for a purpose, your child has also been created uniquely. From the start you will begin to recognize strengths, gifts, likes and abilities that are unique to this child. What is even more amazing is that God has chosen you to parent this child. Your motherhood is not an accident. You were selected to be the steward of this child of God. Though it may initially seem an impossible task, remember God does not give you a responsibility without making you adequate for the task.

Today, you may not feel ready to raise this son or daughter of God. If so, take a deep breath and remember all you are called to do today is to meet today's needs. As your child grows, so will you. Each milestone you mark for your child is also a milestone for you. Before long you will look back and wonder when it happened that you became so patient, or kind, or selfless, or giving, or honest, or loving. The truth is, your children will help you become the woman God created you to be and you will help your children prepare to fulfill the role God has set aside for them.

Letting Go

One of the most amazing things about giving birth is the way your body, the skin in which you live, directs the entire show. The uterus contracts, the cervix opens, the baby descends all without your brain deciding any of it needed to happen. You will not be in control. Labor may begin fast and hard, or labor may slowly build over a day or two. You may suddenly have a strong urge to push or you may slowly have a gentle urge to push. You do not get to choose.

What can be even your normal responses to the work your body is doing may not be considered polite. Some women fear behaving unacceptably during labor. You may get red in the face and your body may feel so hot you need to remove your clothing. You may vomit. You may poop. You may make the same faces and noises you make during sex.

The strong forces moving your baby into the world is your body, yet some women fear feeling helpless or powerless. Your eyes may close and you may not be able to tell people what you need or want. You may not even realize anyone else is in the room with you. That is real labor. But labor does not happen if you are not willing to give up control of your body for the few hours it takes to give birth.

What do you need to allow your body to do the things it needs to do to labor? How can you put aside your pride or need to control the image others have of you? What helps you trust that God made your body adequate to perform this work? Are you ready to let go of control long enough to let your body take over and welcome your child into this world?

Scripture Insight

As you read through the following passages, pay attention to these questions:

1. What are the overall reactions to giving birth?
2. How is the greeting of a child influenced by culture and society?
3. How is the greeting of a child influenced by events in the mother's life?
4. What part does the father play in greeting the child?

Genesis 4:1-2
Genesis 4:1:17
Genesis 4:25
Genesis 16:15
Genesis 19:31-38
Genesis 21:1-5
Genesis 25:21-26
Genesis 29: 31-30:12
Genesis 30:21
Genesis 35:16-18
Genesis 38:27-30
Exodus 1:15-22
Exodus 2:14
Exodus 2:22
1 Chronicles 4:9
1 Samuel 1
1 Samuel 4:19
2 Samuel 12:15-24
Judges 13
Ruth 4:13
2 Kings 4:8-17
1 Samuel 4:19
Hosea 1
Matthew 1:18-25
Luke 1:57-58

To Pray About

In what ways do you fear you will fail as a parent?
In what ways do you feel prepared to parent?
What do you need to do to be ready to let go?

Unit Three
Greeting Baby

My Thoughts...

Unique Creations

Psalm 57:2

Psalm 139:14

John 19:25-27

Romans 12:6-8

Philippians 2:3-8

Unit Four
Choosing With Love

Overview

The options you have for labor will sometimes present themselves with a definite "answer." But just as frequently there will be no obvious right or wrong choice. It is the right and responsibility of the parents to make decisions that will affect the health of their child. You should never feel forced, coerced or manipulated into any decision.

When choosing how to handle labor, or when making any decision that will affect your child, a key point of stewardship will be loving your child with the sacrificial love Jesus modeled for us. Your decisions should be made focused on meeting the needs of and protecting your baby. This means your baby's health should be your highest priority.

There is no cookie cutter answer for what a labor should look like when the health of the baby is the highest priority. You will simply make the best decisions you can with the information you have at the time. That may mean you have exactly the birth you want, or you may not want the choices you know are right for labor.

Discussion Points

- ✓ There are a wide variety of options available for use as comfort measures that do not add risk for baby, and may actually help progress labor.
- ✓ Medicines are a tool. They are neither evil nor good. Depending on what is happening they can help or hinder you. Use them wisely.
- ✓ The attitude in which you make a decision may be more important than the decision you make. Whatever you decide to do, are you doing it out of a servant's heart?
- ✓ When seeking information, be sure to ask the question you want answered. A vague question will get a vague answer.
- ✓ Before you can build your birth plan, you will need to do some searching in your heart to discover what is most important for you.

Personal Study

- ❧ Ask some friends or relatives how they made their decisions about birth options. What sources of information did they use? In what ways were they satisfied? What would they change for their next labor, why?
- ❧ Read Bible stories that let you see an individual making decisions such as Cain (Genesis 4:1-16), Nehemiah (Nehemiah 1) or Daniel (Daniel 1). What good or bad patterns do you see?
- ❧ Make a list of questions to discuss with your doctor or midwife.

Scripture Checklist
- ❏ Luke 9:23-24
- ❏ 1 John 3:16
- ❏ Philippians 2:3-8
- ❏ John 13:34-35
- ❏ John 15:12
- ❏ 1 John 4:7-11
- ❏ Matthew 7:12
- ❏ Proverbs 14:8
- ❏ Psalm 20:4
- ❏ Proverbs 2:6
- ❏ Galatians 5:22
- ❏
- ❏
- ❏
- ❏

Suggested Readings

Lord of Birth
Love

Christian Childbirth Handbook
Options for Labor

Birthing Naturally Web site
Options for Childbirth

Unit Four
Choosing With Love
My Thoughts...

Options for Labor

Use this list to help you investigate your options and keep track of which ones are best for your labor. You do not need to include everything in a written birth plan; only include those issues about which you have a preference.

Starting or Speeding Labor
Spontaneous ○Up to 42 weeks ○Beyond 42 weeks
Self Induced ○Walk ○Enema ○Castor Oil ○Nipple Stimulation ○Acupressure
Medically Induced ○Prostaglandin Gel ○IV Oxytocin ○Amniotomy ○Misoprostol

Monitoring Labor
Intermittent ○Fetoscope ○Doptone ○External Monitor ○Telemetry
Continuous ○External Monitor ○Internal Monitor

Hydration
IV Fluids ○Saline Lock ○NPO (No liquids by mouth)
Clear Liquids ○Popsicles ○Ice Chips ○Lollipops ○Broth ○Tea ○Sodas
According to Thirst ○Limited to clear liquids ○No limit

Pain Relief
Relaxation Techniques ○Breathing ○Visualization ○Focus ○Massage ○Vocalization
Narcotic ○Only if requested ○Offer as soon as possible
Epidural/Spinal ○As Soon As Possible ○When Requested ○Walking/Light

Comfort Items and Techniques
Environment ○Lighting ○Temperature ○Music ○Fresh Air ○Own Clothing/Bedding
Water ○Labor Tub ○Birth Pool ○Shower
Massage Tools ○Tennis Ball ○Rolling Pin ○Heating Pad ○Ice Pack ○Lotion

Positions
Upright ○Walking ○Lunging ○Leaning on Wall/Person ○Sitting on Ball ○Rocking Chair
Hands and Knees ○With Ball ○On Bed ○Pelvic Rocking ○Chest to Floor
Reclining ○On side ○Recliner Chair

Pushing
Positions ○Squatting ○Standing ○Hands and Knees ○Reclining
Duration ○Spontaneous ○Directed ○Prolonged
Perineal Care ○Support ○Massage ○Compresses ○Positioning ○Episiotomy

Cesarean
Support ○Partner ○Doula ○Family Members
Anesthesia ○Epidural ○Spinal ○General
Environment ○Describe Events ○Video/Photos ○Baby and Mom Together for Recovery

Baby Care
Cord Cutting ○Partner ○Mother ○Family Members ○Wait until stops pulsing
Temperature Regulation ○Mother's Abdomen ○Warming Unit
Procedures ○Delay Procedures ○Vaccinations ○Circumcision ○First Bath ○Footprints
Nursery ○Rooming In ○Partner Rooming In ○Nursery on Request ○Pacifier / Bottle

Other options available at your birthplace:

Unit Four
Choosing With Love

Facing the Facts

There are many topics in the field of obstetrics that experts disagree about. To better understand some of the issues you face as a parent, choose a few topics that are important to you, and create a list of the pros and cons for those procedures or techniques. Some examples may be

> Episiotomy
> Elective Cesarean Section
> Routine use of Electronic Fetal Monitors
> Routine use of Intravenous Fluids
> Oxytocin for labor augmentation or induction

You may find information in magazine articles, medical journals, newspapers, internet articles or books. As you review the literature, begin to think of questions you will want to ask of your health care professional. Also make sure you can answer questions such as:

- What is an appropriate use of the intervention?
- What are the risks of this intervention?
- What alternatives are available?
- How might this intervention be prevented?

Use this space to keep brief notes:

Topic:

Pro

Con

Topic:

Pro

Con

Topic:

Pro

Con

My Thoughts...

**Unit Four
Choosing With Love
My Thoughts...**

Making Decisions About Interventions

Each intervention has specific benefits and risks. Most situations have more than one way you can handle them. Your job is to determine how to handle each situation so the benefits of your decision outweigh the risks.

What is the importance of knowing the answers to the following questions?

Why is this being recommended?

What do you hope will be accomplished by using this intervention?

What are the risks of using this intervention?

What is the next step if this does not work?

What are my other options and what are their risks?

Discussion Questions:
What are some ways to get the answers to these questions?
How do these ways compare to each other?

Handling Medication Side Effects

Although medications can help women during labor, they sometimes cause unwanted side effects. Not every woman will experience every side effect from a medication, and there is no way to know which side effects you may experience. For that reason, it is best to be familiar with a variety of ways to manage the most common side effects.

Itching

Cool cloths on skin
Cold packs on skin
Naloxone iv (reduces pain relief)
Avoid fentanyl in the next dose (reduces pain relief)
Diphenhydramine (makes you sleepy)

Shivering

Warm IV fluid
Warm blankets
Complete Relaxation/Hypnotic state

Nausea/Vomiting

Cool cloths or ice to forehead or neck
Peppermint lozenge
Peppermint, citrus or lavender essential oil
Fennel or ginger tea
Sugar water
Mouthwash
Pharmacological Relief

Urinary Retention

Empty bladder before administration
Try toilet/bedpan after 1 hour
Turn on trickling water
Be patient
Peppermint essential oil in the bedpan/toilet (1 drop)
Catheterization

Inadequate Pain Relief

Wait 20 minutes for full effect of medication
Turn to side of most pain (gravity helps)
Try to pinpoint where you feel pain
Call the anesthesiologist and explain what you feel
Use breathing and focusing techniques

Discussion Questions:

Which methods are most agreeable to you?
How can you be ready to use these during labor?

Unit Four
Choosing With Love
My Thoughts...

Unit Four
Choosing With Love
My Thoughts...

Labor Story One

Read this story, paying attention to the choices made by the family. Answer the questions at the end of the story.

I was on the phone with a friend after work when my water broke. No contractions, no sound, just suddenly sitting in a puddle of water. We quickly put our bags in the car and my husband drove to the hospital.

I had changed clothes before we left, but was soaked again by the time we arrived at the hospital. After I got into the bed, the nurse attached a monitor and asked me the standard questions. I still had no contractions.

Our doctor came by to see me around 9:00 p.m. When he checked, I was two to three centimeters dilated but still not having any contractions. The doctor knew we wanted a natural birth, so recommended I walk around to see if labor would start. I walked around for two hours and still had no contractions. My doctor came back to discuss some blood work with me. He informed me the results meant I should be induced now instead of waiting for labor to start on its own.

The nurse attached IV synthetic oxytocin, and within five minutes I had very painful contractions. I used the breathing and relaxation techniques I had learned until 4:30 in the morning when I asked for some pain medication. The nurse checked me before giving me a narcotic, and I was 4 centimeters.

The narcotic made me feel drunk but was not doing anything for the pain I felt. The nurse checked me again at 6:30, I was 8 centimeters that time. She said if I wanted an epidural I needed to have one now or it would be too late. I told her no, and was upset that she would say that to me.

I felt the urge to push by 7:30. The nurse checked me, and I was fully dilated. I pushed as hard as I could, and my baby was born at 9:10.

1. Where might you have made the same decisions?

2. Where might you have made different decisions?

3. What are possible outcomes of decisions you would make?

4. What other options are available, even if you would not choose them?

5. What are the possible outcomes of the other options?

Labor Story Two

Read this story, paying attention to the choices made by the family. Answer the questions at the end of the story.

I just expected my baby was going to be born on my due date. But the due date came and went without any signs of labor. A week after my due date I was a physical and emotional wreck. I could not believe how much weight I had gained, my whole body felt swollen, I could not wear my shoes. I broke down and cried to my doctor, so he decided I should be induced.

I arrived at the hospital at 6:00 am, filled out the paperwork and was officially admitted by 8:00. As part of the admitting, a nurse anesthetist came to explain the pain medication options to me. I was very opposed to anyone putting a needle in my back, and how bad could labor be anyway?

My induction started around 9, and my water was spontaneously broken by 10. I just remember the contractions being so strong and the pressure being severe. I would walk back and forth between the bathroom and the bed, dragging the IV with me.

By 11 I was in tears, begging for an epidural. The nurse told me I could not have an epidural until I was 4 centimeters. As I was trying to convince her to check my dilation, I started to have an urge to push. She seemed shocked and quickly checked me. She felt my baby's head and called for my doctor. She gave me a shot to help me relax, which I thought was wonderful. My baby was born at 12:30.

1. What evidence can you see that tells you this might be a fast labor?

2. Can you identify the stages of labor for this mother?

3. What options did this woman choose to use?

4. What options were available to this woman that she did not use?

5. What effects might those options have had?

6. Where might you have made different decisions?

Unit Four
Choosing With Love
My Thoughts...

Unit Four
Choosing With Love
My Thoughts...

Discussing Options with your Caregiver

Some women get nervous when they talk to their caregiver. This nervousness is unnecessary. Your caregiver is working for you. If you are dissatisfied with the quality of work she is doing for you, hire someone else.

Plan

- ✓ Research the topics that are most important to you.
- ✓ Keep a list of questions and issues you want to discuss with your caregiver. Take it with you to your appointments so you do not forget anything.

Discuss

- ✓ Let your caregiver know at the beginning of the appointment that you want to ask a few questions; if she forgets, gently remind her before the appointment is done. Be sure to let your caregiver know you are interested in her thoughts and opinions of the options in general and in your case specifically.
- ✓ When possible take something you have read on the subject with you. Share with your caregiver the sources of information you have on the subject and why they have led you to the conclusions you have made.
- ✓ Ask your caregiver if she has any literature on the subject, or if she can recommend a book or web site so you can keep researching the issue. If your caregiver disagrees with your views on a subject, let her know you will continue to research the subject and want to talk to her about it again at your next appointment. This will give her time to do some more research and gather information to help you make a decision. It also lets her know that this issue is important to you.

Review

- ✓ Consider the information you received from your caregiver and any new research she suggested.
- ✓ Maintain a list of questions and ideas to share at your next appointment.

How to Ask Questions

When asking questions, ask the specific questions you want the answered. Asking, "How often do you do episiotomies?" will give you the answer, "I only do them when necessary." Instead ask,

> "How many of your clients need episiotomies?"
> "Under what circumstances do you recommend an episiotomy?"
> "What techniques do you use to help keep perineal skin intact?"

Write three questions you will ask of your caregiver at your next visit.

1.

2.

3.

My choices

You have explored the normal process of labor, comfort measures and the options available. You have probably begun making decisions about how you want to handle labor. Complete these statements.

1. If everything goes perfect, I would like my labor to be...

2. If safety concerns arise before labor begins, I would like to...

3. If safety concerns arise during labor, I would like to...

4. If my comfort plan is inadequate during labor, I would like to...

5. To increase my chances of having the labor I desire, I am...

Unit Four
Choosing With Love
My Thoughts...

**Unit Four
Choosing With Love
My Thoughts...**

Epidural Assessment

Mark each statement as true or false, then turn to page 62 to check your answers.

1. An epidural removes the pain while allowing labor to continue normally.
2. Epidurals are the most effective medications for managing pain during labor.
3. An epidural will remove all the pain of labor.
4. It may take up to an hour to receive relief after choosing to have an epidural.
5. You can still walk with an epidural.
6. An epidural can allow a woman to sleep during labor.
7. Epidurals do not affect the baby.
8. Epidural administration requires you to sit still even during contractions.
9. Epidurals improve satisfaction with labor.
10. Epidurals are not always readily available.
11. There is a cut-off after which you will not be allowed to have an epidural.
12. You can have an epidural with a midwife.
13. You need to stop an epidural for pushing.
14. Epidurals are used for cesarean surgical births.
15. Epidurals reduce the chances you will tear or need an episiotomy.
16. An epidural can affect your baby's heart rate.
17. Epidurals speed labor.
18. Women with epidurals often need a catheter to urinate.
19. Epidurals do not increase the rate of cesarean surgery.
20. There is no standard dosage/technique for epidural medication use during labor.
21. Epidurals cause headaches.
22. Epidurals require continuous fetal monitoring.
23. There are no side effects with epidural.
24. Women with an epidural need to change positions regularly to prevent a "window" of pain on one side.
25. You cannot use an epidural if you have had a previous cesarean.

Unit Four
Choosing With Love
My Thoughts...

What Will I Choose?

I have a choice to make. For the next few hours I will be engaged in the most demanding work I have ever done. But since this is the most important work I will ever do…

I will do it with love…
This is my baby's birth day. It is not about my needs, my desires, my hopes or my feelings. Because I love my child, I will put myself in God's hands so I can concentrate on giving my baby the birth he needs.

I will do it with joy…
Although I may feel temptation to wallow in self-pity, I will be thankful for every contraction. I will rejoice that every contraction brings me one step closer to the moment I have waited for so long.

I will do it with peace…
I will not battle my body or my baby. I will simply allow my baby to use my body as an entrance point for life.

I will do it with patience…
I will not lose sight of the fact that my sense of time may be skewed, and what feels like a lifetime is really only a few hours of waiting. I will not make decisions that put myself or my baby at risk simply to shorten the time I must wait.

I will do it with kindness…
I will be kind to my baby; she is alone, and she may be frightened. I will not allow myself to benefit by putting her at risk.

I will do it with goodness…
I will not let myself give into the temptation to use labor as an excuse to be rude, angry, mean, hurtful, lazy or prideful. This is my first opportunity to teach my baby about relationships.

I will do it with faithfulness…
I will not question God's love or goodness as I pass through this time of trial. I will not let my actions or reactions be a reason for others to question my love or goodness.

I will do it with gentleness…
As I welcome my baby, may he only hear my voice raised in joy; may she only see my arms raised in praise; and may he only feel the touch of love.

I will do it with self control…
I will not allow myself to lower my standards simply because I am in labor. I will continue to strive for excellent character regardless of the challenges.

In a few moments, my baby will arrive. For the next few hours, I will be exposed to labor's demands. It is now that I must make a choice.

Discussion Question:
How would you interpret Galatians 5:22-23?

Unit Four
Choosing With Love

My Thoughts...

Hearing the Voice of God

Sometimes the voice of God is as loud as the thunder, you know clearly what you should do. Sometimes the voice of God is as soft as a gentle breeze; unless you quiet yourself and listen, you will not hear it. If you are not sure where God is leading you for this birth, consider trying a new way to listen for his voice. There are as many ways to quiet yourself before God as there are unique people he has created.

You could go for a walk in the woods, on the beach, through the fields, up a mountain or in the heart of the city.

You could sit silently under a tree, at the edge of the ocean, in a crowded coffee shop or your own bedroom.

You might need to stop working through your to-do list, or begin a project you have been putting off.

You might want to open your mouth to pour out your heart, keep your mouth closed for a while or use your voice to sing worship and praise.

You may need to begin letting others serve you, or begin serving others.

You may want to read a different version of the Bible or listen to a recorded Bible.

Explore new ways to spend time with God. Enjoy yourself as you learn about all the unique voices he uses to speak with you.

Making Good Use of Your Tools

Medicine and other health technology are tools. They are neither good nor evil. Depending on how labor is progressing, they can either help or hinder the process. Use them wisely.

The key to making good use of your tools is to be aware of the risks and benefits. Using a tool that adds minimal benefit while increasing risk to you or your baby is unwise. At best, tools should be used to decrease the risk, at minimum they should not add risk.

In general, there is more than one way to handle any labor challenge. A tired mother may benefit from a narcotic, but she may also benefit from a massage, a warm bath, changing positions or deep relaxation between contractions. Once you know what tools may be beneficial, you can look at the associated risks.

One way to maintain the lowest risk possible is to always use the tools with the lowest risk first. If that does not work, you can always try something with more risk. Give yourself adequate time to try low-risk tools before moving on to higher risk tools. Your goal should always be to keep the risk as low as possible for both you and your baby.

Epidural Assessment:

All the even numbered questions are true. All the odd numbered statements are false. For more information about epidural pain relief for labor, please see the Birthing Naturally web site at www.birthingnaturally.net.

Unit Four
Choosing With Love

Scripture Insight

As you read through the verses from the scripture checklist on page 51, meditate on these questions.

1. What does it mean that God loves you?

2. What does it mean to love God?

3. Explain why Christ is our example of love.

4. Describe what life is like when loving God is your first priority.

5. In what ways do you feel pregnancy can display your love for God?

6. In what ways do you feel giving birth can display your love for God?

To Pray About

In the past, how have you been sure you are following God's plan?
What options for labor do you feel uncomfortable about? Why?
Seek the wisdom of God for making decisions.

My Thoughts...

Wisdom

Proverbs 2:6

Proverbs 16:3

Psalm 119:148

Isaiah 58:11

1 Timothy 4:14

Unit Five
Labor Challenges

Scripture Checklist
- ☐ Isaiah 55:8-9
- ☐ Proverbs 18:13
- ☐ John 8:32
- ☐ James 3:17
- ☐ John 14:27
- ☐ James 1:2-4
- ☐ Psalm 4:8
- ☐ Psalm 29:11
- ☐ Deuteronomy 31:6
- ☐
- ☐
- ☐
- ☐

Overview

The truth is sometimes hard to see. How can you be sure that what you are deciding is the best option unless you understand the truth about what is happening? There are many variations of the normal, healthy labor. You may be experiencing something that is not average, and still be completely healthy. Knowing what signals a problem and being able to adjust for that problem are key components of stewardship.

There are several ways in which you may be challenged during labor. It is not enough to just recognize the challenge; you will need to be able to respond to the challenge effectively. The goal of this unit is to learn to differentiate between a birth emergency and a normal variation of labor; and how to respond to each.

While preparing to make wise decisions, it is possible to over-prepare. Birth emergencies are very rare, so your chances of experiencing one are small. It is possible to struggle with trusting God instead of your knowledge. Not only should you aim to make good decisions during a challenge, but also to continue experiencing the peace of God during the storm.

Discussion Points

- ✓ Some challenges will present themselves before labor begins, giving you a chance to make changes during pregnancy.
- ✓ Using medical interventions when a challenge arises will make changes. Sometimes the changes are what you want, and other times they are not.
- ✓ God has a purpose for your labor, and he will teach you something from labor. However, you may not discover what it is until months later.
- ✓ Even if you make changes, you may not be able to end a labor challenge. You can only respond to what is happening; you cannot control your labor.
- ✓ There are a number of reasons why a woman may experience a challenge in labor. It is not necessarily a sign of a lack of faith.

Personal Study

- ☙ Make a list of your gifts and strengths. How can you use those to overcome any challenges?
- ☙ Talk to family and friends about their labor and birth challenges. What options did they choose? How did those options change labor?
- ☙ Reread the story of your favorite Bible character. What can you learn from the stories of challenges in the Bible?

Suggested Readings

Lord of Birth
Faith

Christian Childbirth Handbook
Labor Challenges

Birthing Naturally Web site
Labor Challenges

Unit Five
Labor Challenges

My Thoughts...

Difficult Spots in Labor

You can expect there will be certain times during labor that will be more difficult than others. Be prepared to handle these occurrences.

Why might the following times be difficult?
What could be done to help the mother through this difficult spot?

Onset of labor

Moving to the hospital

During examination

Beginning of transition

Beginning of pushing

Crowning

Discussion Question:
What does it mean to persevere through a trial?
How do you, as a Christian, overcome a challenge?

Variations of Normal Before Labor

You may know about some challenges before labor begins, allowing you time to make changes.

What is challenging in each of these situations?
Which challenges are you facing?
What options do you have for managing your challenges?

Breech Position

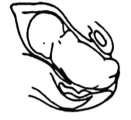

Transverse Position

Gestational Diabetes

Group B Strep

Overdue/ Postmaturity

History of Abuse

Advanced Maternal Age

Sixth or more time giving birth

Multiple Pregnancy

Pre-eclampsia

Obesity

Unit Five
Labor Challenges
My Thoughts...

Unit Five
Labor Challenges
My Thoughts...

Variations of Normal During Labor

Some challenges you will not know about until labor begins. What are these challenges, and what options do you have if they occur?

Discouraged Mother

Fast Labor

Posterior Baby

Ascynclitic Baby

Premature Rupture of Membranes

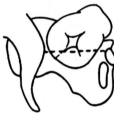

Slow Progress

Birth Emergencies

A birth emergency is not a normal variation of labor. It is an emergency situation in which your baby's life is in danger. True birth emergencies are rare. What are each of these emergencies, and what can be done about them?

Fetal Distress

Placental Previa

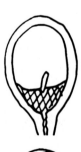

Placental Abruption

Umbilical Cord Prolapse

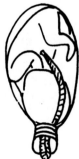

Hemorrhage

Handling Labor Challenges

Knowing how to handle a labor challenge requires understanding what is happening, and how your body may react to the various options. To help you organize this information, take some time to make a Venn diagram.

1. Determine if what is happening is a normal variation of labor, is a variation that may signal a potential complication, or is a dangerous situation for mother and/or baby. Place the challenges in the appropriate part of the diagram.

2. Select a response to the challenge, such as induction, position change or surgical birth. Place the response in the appropriate part of the diagram.

3. In the overlap between response and challenges, write what you may expect from using this response in this situation.

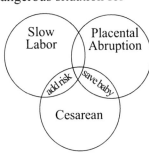

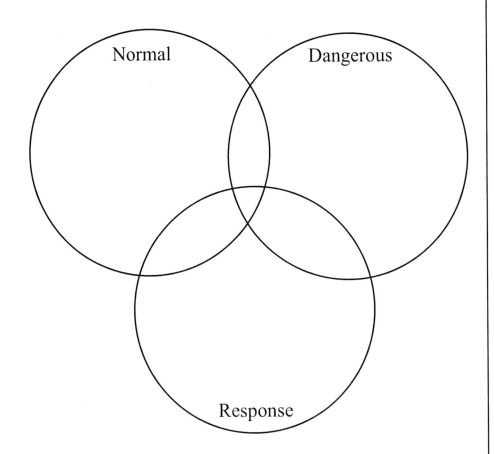

Discussion Question:
Why is it important to understand the potential effects of the options for responding to labor challenges?

Unit Five
Labor Challenges

My Thoughts...

**Unit Five
Labor Challenges
My Thoughts...**

Cesarean Surgery

Some reasons for cesarean birth include...

If a cesarean is done, these procedures will happen...

If a cesarean is done, these procedures might happen...

If a cesarean is done, these options may be available. Talk to your doctor or midwife to find out what additional options are available.

When to start the surgery

When to have family join you

Medication used

Support person with you at all times

Photo or video documentation

Surgeon describes events

Immediate breast feeding

Someone with baby at all times

Labor Challenges Role Play

How might a mother handle the following challenging labor situations?

Mother appears to be in early labor. She is not using any comfort measures yet, can still talk and move through contractions and is in good spirits. With the next contraction she feels a trickle of fluid from her vagina.

Contractions began as a dull backache. Now that they are regular and building in intensity, the backache is becoming more painful. Mother does not want to walk during a contraction and is in pain between contractions.

The due date came and went 6 days ago. At the visit to the midwife, she recommends the mother be induced.

Labor started suddenly. After just two hours of contractions, the mother is in active labor, breathing hard and working to relax through the 60 second long contractions. The mother says she needs something.

The mother has had contractions on and off for about two weeks. Contractions began again yesterday, but are not intense enough for the mother to have to do anything with them.

At the 35 week checkup, the midwife told the mother the baby is in a breech position.

The mother is feeling light contractions when suddenly her water breaks with a gush of fluid. As she dries herself off she realizes she feels something stuck to her leg. She is concerned it may be the umbilical cord.

Unit Five
Labor Challenges
My Thoughts...

Unit Five
Labor Challenges

My Thoughts...

Knowing the Truth

There is a reason Jesus said the truth will set us free; we live in a world surrounded by lies. We receive messages daily that we are not good enough, smart enough, strong enough...just not enough. None of this is true. God has made each of us adequate for the tasks he has for us. Yet the lies continue to bombard our hearts and minds.

In addition to the lies about who we are, we are told lies about the way the world works. Messages about what is or is not sin; what is or is not good for us and even what is or is not normal during childbirth. We are told everything will be perfect if we know this one thing; hire this one doctor; go to this one birth center; use this one comfort technique. Yet nothing we do can guarantee perfection.

The process of labor is beautifully simple, yet relies on a complex balance of hormones, movements, contractions and time. Sometimes the changes we make help this intricate system to work more efficiently. Other times, adding a new component to the mix can throw off a system that is otherwise working well. You will find it helpful to understand the benefits and risks of any tool available to you so you can understand the changes it may bring.

Even with the best preparation and the best labor team you may still face a challenge in labor. Making changes in response to a challenge may not always give you the desired result. Although certain techniques can be effective, they are not going to be effective every time they are used. It can take two or three tries before you find what works best.

Even if you make appropriate changes, you may not be able to end a labor challenge. You can only respond to what is happening; you cannot control your labor. God has a purpose for your labor, even if you do not discover what it is until much later.

Having Peace

In the midst of uncertainty, you can have peace.

Do not confuse safety with peace. Peace is not having everything perfect. Peace is not an uneventful labor. Peace is not the absence of fear or concern. Peace is trusting in God in the midst of a storm, in the middle of uncertainty, while you are afraid.

When Jonathan approached the Philistines in 1 Samuel 14, he understood he could be walking to his death, but he had peace in his decision because he knew whether he lived or died in battle was up to God.

In Matthew 8:23-27 (Mark 4:35-41; Luke 8:22-25), the disciples in the boat with Jesus were frightened as the storm raged, but felt peace when Jesus calmed the storm. It was not their safety that changed, only the appearance of safety. They were safe in the midst of the storm even if they did not understand. The ultimate authority of God can bring peace in the midst of your labor challenges.

Unit Five
Labor Challenges

My Thoughts...

God's Strength and Safety

1 Chronicles 16:11

Psalm 4:8

Psalm 18:32

Psalm 29:11

Scripture Insight

Read Amos 4 and John 9

1. Describe the potential impact of the challenges God sent to the people.

2. What reason does God give for sending these challenges.

3. What conclusions can you draw about the people's reactions?

4. What reason does Jesus give for the man's blindness.

5. Describe the challenges of having been blind.

6. Explain why the man being healed was a challenge to the Pharisees.

7. What challenges have you faced in your life?

To Pray About

How does experiencing a labor challenge test your faith in God?
How does experiencing a labor challenge strengthen your faith in God?
In what ways is your spiritual life reflected by the type of labor you have?

Unit Six
Birth Planning

Overview

This week you will be putting your thoughts, opinions and decisions about labor into a written format that can be shared with your health care professionals. As you work through putting your ideas on paper, you will have one last opportunity to do a heart-check. Are you making decisions from a pure heart devoted only to God? Are you making decisions from a heart of fear? Are you making decisions from a heart devoted to self?

Any impurities in your heart will cause you not only problems in your relationship with Christ, but also in your labor. Fear, anxiety and worry have a negative effect on a laboring body. Work to remove them before labor begins.

Discussion Points

- ✓ A birth plan is not a script that is to be followed exactly. It is a set of guidelines to help those with you understand how they can be of most service to you.
- ✓ Your birth plan is just as important before labor begins as it is once you are in labor.
- ✓ God's plan for your labor may not be the same as yours. Even with the best health habits and making the best decisions, your labor may not go exactly as you had planned.
- ✓ Writing your birth plan can serve as a heart check for you to ensure you are maintaining the purity of worshiping God alone. Be aware of any fears or concerns that still plague you.
- ✓ There is just as much trust that happens while you wait for labor as there is happening once labor begins.

Personal Study

- ❧ Talk to other families who have recently had a baby. Did they write a birth plan? How helpful was writing the plan? How did they choose what to put in it? How did they use the plan before and during labor?
- ❧ Read a few sample birth plans. You can find some on the internet or by asking birth professionals in your area. Make a list of the things you like and do not like in the samples you see.
- ❧ Read about Paul's journeys in Acts 13-28. Although he had plans, his journeys did not always turn out as he anticipated. What can you learn from the way Paul handled the challenges he faced?

Scripture Checklist
- ❏ Matthew 15:16-20
- ❏ Luke 6:45
- ❏ Jeremiah 17:9
- ❏ Deuteronomy 8:2
- ❏ Psalm 26:2
- ❏ Psalm 139:23
- ❏ 2 Corinthians 13:5
- ❏ Galatians 6:4
- ❏ Proverbs 3:25-26
- ❏
- ❏
- ❏
- ❏

Suggested Readings
Lord of Birth
Holiness

Christian Childbirth Handbook
Birth Planning

Birthing Naturally Web site
Birth Planning

**Unit Six
Birth Planning**

My Thoughts...

Writing a Birth Plan

Before you begin, you need to know what it is you are writing. Answer these questions in your own words.

What is a birth plan?

What are common misunderstandings about birth plans?

What options may be available for a birth plan?

What options do you feel most strongly about?

Regarding the options you feel most strongly about:

- Are they available at your birth place and with your caregiver?

- Does it make sense given your health and other circumstances?

- How have you started talking about your choices with your caregiver?

Discussion Question:
How will you know when your birth plan is the right plan for you?

Planning With the End in Mind

Think of the way you would like to describe your labor experience after your baby is born. Try to write a word or phrase you would want to use to describe labor for each letter of the alphabet.

A
B
C
D
E
F
G
H
I
J
K
L
M
N
O
P
Q
R
S
T
U
V
W
X
Y
Z

Discussion Question:
What will help you achieve your ideal labor?
What can prevent you from achieving your ideal labor?

Unit Six
Birth Planning

My Thoughts...

Unit Six
Birth Planning

My Thoughts...

Theories of Managing Labor Pain

Can you explain each theory?
How you can use the principles to promote comfort during labor?

Gate Control Theory
Large Nerve Fibers: Pressure, non-damaging heat and cold,
Small Nerve Fibers: Pain, extreme heat and cold, light touch
Habituation occurs about 15-20 minutes into a large-nerve strategy.

Hawthorne Effect
A person performs better when receiving specialized attention.

Endorphin Levels
Rise as labor progresses. Stop rising when medication is used.

Confidence
One of the most important factors in a woman's ability to handle labor is her confidence in her ability to handle labor.

Fear-Tension-Pain Cycle

Dr. Grantly Dick-Read coined the term Fear-Tension-Pain cycle to describe a common experience in labor. Explain each step of the cycle.

Fear:

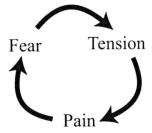

Tension:

Pain:

How does this apply to you specifically? We are all uniquely created, with different strengths and struggles. Our personalities and the way we cope with challenges are all different. So, how can you stop the cycle if you...

Experience Fear?

Experience Tension?

Experience Pain?

Unit Six
Birth Planning
My Thoughts...

Unit Six
Birth Planning

My Thoughts...

Cultural Beliefs

Are you aware that many of your beliefs about childbirth may be due to cultural attitudes rather than the truth about birth? In the following examples, you will be faced with a potential change in the "rules" for giving birth. Consider the ways attitudes and beliefs about birth would need to be changed if the potential change were real.

Currently, pain medication is available for any woman to use during labor and over 70% of American women use an epidural during vaginal birth. How might cultural beliefs and attitudes about birth need to change if pain medications were only available for women undergoing surgical birth?

Currently, over 40% of American women have induction recommended to them. How might cultural beliefs and attitudes about birth need to change if induction were not available?

Currently, many women have their health care costs paid for by insurance. How might cultural belief and attitudes about birth change if families were required to pay for their own maternity fees?

Currently, 90% of American women hire a surgeon to attend them during labor. How might cultural belief and attitudes about birth change if surgeons were only available for surgical birth?

Now that you have confronted some of the cultural biases about giving birth, try to think of more areas in which your birth beliefs may be culturally biased.

Unit Six
Birth Planning
My Thoughts...

Opinions

While you may not understand everything there is to know about giving birth, you are already forming opinions based on the information you have learned. It is time to express your opinions and begin discussing them with others.

Not only do you have opinions, but you are making decisions based on the opinions you hold. Take some time to explore your opinions, and what they mean to your birth preparation.

For each statement, state if you agree or disagree. This is not a true or false quiz, it is simply an expression of your opinions. Take each statement as it is written, whatever it means to you. Pay special attention to the statements you find you have the most difficulty answering, God may be trying to teach you something.

- Pregnancy is a healthy time in a woman's life.

- Giving birth is painful.

- The female body is designed to give birth.

- Epidurals make labor better.

- Birth is a private husband/wife event.

- A laboring woman should be attended by women.

- Hospitals are safe environments for babies to be born.

- The home is a safe environment for babies to be born.

- It takes great strength to give birth.

- Natural birth is the healthiest birth.

- Elective cesarean should be offered to all women.

- Elective induction should be offered to all women.

- Every woman should have a doula.

- Bottle feeding is a good option for mothers.

If you have difficulty expressing your opinions try to figure out why. Write your reasons here.

Unit Six
Birth Planning

My Thoughts...

Wise Decision

For each scenario, answer these questions.

What are the risks to the suggestion?
What are other options that may be available?
What are potential risks to the other options?
What coaching techniques could be used in this situation?

1. My water broke three hours ago, but contractions have not started yet. When I called my doctor she said I should come to the hospital for antibiotics and to start an induction.

2. My baby has been in breech position at the last three appointments. My doctor says if the baby does not move by next week I will have to have a cesarean because if I get any closer to my due date I may start labor.

3. After I am admitted to the hospital, I realize I am hungry. The nurse informs me I am only allowed ice chips and water. She says if I take medication after eating I could vomit, which may be dangerous.

4. I have been having very strong contractions for the last 5 hours, but my dilation has not changed. My doctor says the baby is probably just too big to fit through my pelvis. He suggested we do a cesarean.

5. I had my first contraction during the 11:00 news, and already at 3:00 am they are 3 minutes apart and I think I may be in transition. The nurse says this is happening too fast, and if I have an epidural the contractions will get easier to handle.

6. After 10 hours of laboring at home, I talked my support into going to the hospital (even though they believed it was too early). The nurse said I was only dilated 2 cm, and that she should call the doctor to order synthetic oxytocin because my body did not seem to be getting anywhere.

7. I am shaking, and can not get comfortable even between contractions. I feel like I am going to be sick, andt I can not do this anymore. The nurse says that she will get something for the pain.

8. I was not expecting the pushing contractions to be so uncomfortable. Every time the contraction starts I throw my head back and scream. The nurse suggests that using stirrups to support my legs may help me.

9. I was certain I was in transition, but suddenly the contractions stopped and I have not had one for twenty minutes. It has been a long labor, and I am glad for the rest, but the nurse says my body must need some help keep labor moving.

10. You look to see the baby's head slowly emerge and notice the doctor grab what looks like scissors. When you ask what she is doing, she says she needs to do an episiotomy or I will tear.

Birth Plan Check-sheet

Here is a birth plan check sheet to help you ensure your birth plan is complete:

Did you include information about:

- ❑ The environment you hope to achieve.
- ❑ Who you do or do not want with you.
- ❑ How you want to manage pain.
- ❑ The pushing positions you want to try.
- ❑ How you prefer to have the labor monitored.
- ❑ How you want to handle normal variations.
- ❑ How you want to handle complications.
- ❑ How you want to handle a possible cesarean.
- ❑ Your choices for care of your newborn?
- ❑ Any other points important to you.

Is your birth plan:

- ❑ Easy to read.
- ❑ Organized with important points at the top.
- ❑ One page.
- ❑ Proofread by someone you trust.
- ❑ Copied, so you can hand them out.
- ❑ Ready to be shared with those who will support you.

Thoughts about your birth plan:

Unit Six
Birth Planning

My Thoughts...

Unit Six
Birth Planning

My Thoughts...

Setting Your Goals

Think for a few minutes about what your ideal labor experience might be. Consider who is with you, where you are and what things are available to you. Imagine how you might handle both the expected and unexpected situations that may arise. Reflect on which of these is the most important to you.

Keeping these things in mind, write out your plans. This will not be a script to be followed exactly, but a sort of calling card to help those with you understand what help you would like during labor.

Writing a birth plan is just as important before labor begins as it is during labor. You should be using it to talk with your midwife about questions you have and options available to you. In this way, you can be sure you will work together to achieve the best labor experience possible.

Understand you may not be able to do anything on your birth plan. Your labor may move too fast for you to try some comfort measures or give birth where you had hoped. Or, you may be able to do everything on your birth plan with a labor that gives you plenty of time to try every comfort technique and ends with a surgical birth using the options you selected in case it was necessary.

Your success in labor is not determined by how strictly you follow your birth plan, but in how effectively your plan is able to meet your needs. For this reason, you must know who you are and what you will need when you write your plan.

A plan that lists everything other people felt was important has little chance of expressing what you will need in labor. A well written plan helps those attending you know who you are and how they can be the most help to you.

God Remains in Control

The book of Judges shows an interesting way in which God works in our plans. Gideon was told to fight, but before God sent him into battle he weaned the army down to about 400 men (Judges 7).

This idea of decreasing the army size goes against our worldly wisdom of the way to achieve victory. In our minds we think, "Give me more God, prove everything will turn out OK and then I will trust you." Gideon had to trust God's seemingly backwards plan would work.

Yet having less was exactly what God needed. It was not the strength of Gideon's army that would win, but the strength of God. Which leads us to an interesting question. What can God wean from your birth plan? Where might you be relying on your power or strength instead of God's?

More importantly, does your plan express what you feel is important, or does it express what is socially acceptable? Was it written with God, or by yourself?

Scripture Insight

Birth was a normal part of life for most people throughout history. Because everyone knew about birth, God was able to use the imagery of birth to help his people understand things they could not see.

The following is a list of verses that use the imagery of birth. As you read the verses, ask yourself:

What is birth being compared to?

What does the analogy say about birth?

John 16:21
Isaiah 42:14
Hosea 13:13
Romans 8:8
Galatians 4:19
2 Kings 19:3
Isaiah 26:17
Isaiah 66:7
Isaiah 66:9
Matthew 24:8
Mark 13:8
Psalm 48:6
Isaiah 13:8
Isaiah 21:3
Jeremiah 4:31
Jeremiah 6:24
Jeremiah 13:21
Jeremiah 22:23
Jeremiah 30:6
Jeremiah 48:41
Micah 4:9-10

To Pray About

What happens when you talk about your birth choices with friends, family, coworkers or your health care provider?

What one thing would you change about being pregnant?

What strength do you bring to this labor?

Unit Six
Birth Planning

My Thoughts...

Planning

Proverbs 15:22

Proverbs 16:9

Proverbs 20:18

Isaiah 55:8

Zechariah 10:1

Haggai 1:5-6

Unit Seven
Self Control

Scripture Checklist
- ❑ Colossians 3:1-2
- ❑ Philippians 3:12-14
- ❑ Proverbs 25:28
- ❑ 2 Peter 1:5-8
- ❑ Joshua 24:15
- ❑ 1 Peter 1:6-7
- ❑ Matthew 6:19-21
- ❑
- ❑
- ❑
- ❑

Overview

You may be more challenged by labor than any other event in your life. It is important to remain focused. However, to accomplish this takes great self-control. Self-control does not mean you are in control of the labor. You cannot control what happens; you can only control how you respond to it.

Self-control is the art of doing what is right even when it is difficult or uncomfortable. It means you are governing your own actions, your responses to labor. It does not mean that you remain rigid or fight what is happening. Instead it means that you are actively working with your body to move through the labor.

Self-control, along with your faith, holiness and love, will help you overcome labor. Be careful how you define overcome. The goal is not to conquer or win, but to get through it with God's help. Labor rehearsals will help you practice your self-control.

Discussion Points

- ✓ You must be in control of your responses to labor, but let God be in control of your labor.
- ✓ Self-control also means "practicing labor" during pregnancy. If you do not practice the comfort measures, you might not be able to use them effectively in labor.
- ✓ The self-control needed is actually a mental or spiritual self-control more than a physical self-control. You must not allow yourself to lose faith in God or the body he has given you.
- ✓ It is nearly impossible for a woman to progress through a normal labor and keep a good attitude. Most women experience a time of "giving up" near the end of labor.
- ✓ God is not so much concerned about achieving your wants and desires for labor as he is with maturing you in a relationship with him.
- ✓ Whether or not labor should hurt is a hotly debated topic even among Christians.

Personal Study

- ✎ Watch some movies or television programs with pregnant women or scenes of birth. What attitudes do these programs portray about pregnancy? What attitudes to these programs portray about giving birth? Why do you agree or disagree with the attitudes they portray?
- ✎ Spend time meditating on Paul and his thorn (2 Corinthians 12), Joseph in jail (Genesis 39-41) or another Biblical trial that seems interesting to you. What do the struggles from the Bible teach you about perseverance?
- ✎ Talk with friends and family about their labor experiences. What did they really like? What do they wish they could do differently and why?

Suggested Readings

Lord of Birth
Propriety

Christian Childbirth Handbook
From Decision to Reality

**Unit Seven
Self Control**

My Thoughts...

Staying Comfortable

How might these items be helpful for you during labor? Which items are available at your birth place, and which ones will you need to bring with you?

Tools for Labor
Birth ball
Hot sock
Massage/aromatherapy oil
Massage tools
Cold pack
Gloves
Relaxing CD's or tapes
Portable tape player
Fan
Washcloths (for cool or heat)
Tennis balls or pool noodle
Pictures for focus
Toothbrush and toothpaste
Sweater or complete change of clothes
Book to read
Kneeling pad
Chapstick
Headache medicine for support people
Water bottle or juice boxes

Try some of these labor tricks during the labor rehearsal. Do you know what each technique is intended to accomplish?

Techniques for Labor
Abdominal Breathing
Aromatherapy
Effleurage
Encouragement
Hip Squeeze
Kneading Massage
The Lift
The Lunge
Massage
Nipple Stimulation
Perineal Massage
Pressure
Progressive Relaxation
Rainbow Technique
Rhythmic Breathing
Stroking
Tug of War
Visualization
Vocalization
Using Water

Massage Techniques to Try

Spend some time trying each of these techniques.

For the Arm:

- Support the arm with one hand and knead the arm with the other. If the arm is large enough you can work with both hands on one side kneading and wringing firmly without hurting.

- Stroke up from elbow and back down in a circle. Try with both hands working opposite (one going up, one going down).

For the Hand:

- Hold her hand palm down and use your other hand to work on each finger separately. Stroke from tip to knuckle, then squeeze finger.

- Hold her hand palm up in one hand and stroke the palm with the heel of your other hand. Push down toward the wrist then glide back.

For the Back:

- Do penetrating circular pressures with your thumbs all over the sacrum (base of the spine). Rest fingers on her hips for support.

- Press deeply with your thumbs into the center of each buttock. This can relieve lower back pain.

For the Foot:

- Support the foot with one hand and stroke the sole firmly with the heel of your other hand.

- Apply deep pressures with your thumbs in a line down the center of the sole to the heel.

For the Face:

- Stroke gently, one hand following the other in a smooth, rhythmic sequence up the forehead into the hairline.

- Place your thumbs on the bridge of the nose. Stroke out to the temples and press gently. Repeat going higher each time.

For the Leg:

- Place your hands on either side of the thigh, fingers facing away from you. Pull your hands up the sides, glide them over the top and down the other side. Work upward from the knee.

- The thighs can take a lot of firm kneading. Work deeply and strongly on the outer thigh and more gently on the inner thigh.

Unit Seven
Self Control

My Thoughts...

**Unit Seven
Self Control**

My Thoughts...

Labor Rehearsal

It is time to practice labor for 20–30 minutes. While you are in labor, you will have contractions that are 60 seconds long and 2 minutes apart.

What does it mean to have 60 second contractions that are two minutes apart?

Please remember this is a serious time to try out different positions and techniques for labor. Practice the first stage positions, not the pushing positions. As you try each position, pay attention to what your support persons are able to do for you. For example, when you are walking your support person has to help hold you up and cannot rub your back; the hands and knees position gives full access to your back but some variations of it may be hard on the arms.

As you go through labor, try to spend time in each of these positions. After the rehearsal, write your reactions to each position.

- Walking and Swaying

- Leaning on a wall or support person

- Sitting

- Using a birth ball

- Sitting backwards on a chair

- Sitting on a toilet

- In hands and knees position

- Dangle position

- Side-lying

- Kneeling with your head down

Unit Seven
Self Control

My Thoughts...

Understanding Your Options

Every option you use will change the way you labor, and the way you manage labor. Answer the following questions to plan for this, and learn ways to work around the most limiting options.

If you could be anywhere and do anything while you labor for your baby, where would you be and what would you do to manage pain, stress or discomfort?

Now, you can do anything, but you have to be in the hospital while you labor. What would you do to manage any stress or discomfort?

Now, you have an IV attached and must move the IV pole with you. What can you do to manage your stress and discomfort?

Now, you have to be monitored and have an IV. These restrict your mobility, but you can still move about 3-4 feet around the monitor. What can you do to manage stress and discomfort?

Now, you have to stay in the bed because you have received a medication that limits your mobility. You also have a monitor and an IV. What can you do while you labor if the medication is effective at blocking your pain?

What can you do during labor if the medication is not effective at blocking your pain?

What can you do if you have consented to a cesarean and are waiting to begin?

Unit Seven
Self Control
My Thoughts...

Labor Role Play

Here is a rehearsal to do with your labor support. Because we learn differently by watching and trying, take turns being the mother and the support person.

The mother will act out (or verbally responds saying how she feels) the scene described.

The support person will decide on and perform appropriate actions for the situation. Appropriate actions may include: words of support or encouragement; physical touch, massage, leading through relaxation, providing for physical needs or simply offering companionship. Which actions by the support person seem like they would be the most helpful?

The mother is in early labor. She has not had to use any comfort measures yet. On this contraction she tenses and squints while holding her breath at the peak of the contraction.

Later in the labor, the mother is feeling contractions mostly as a strong back ache.

Now the mother's slow breathing becomes tense-sounding and strained.

The mother seems to be in active labor. She is moaning, tensing, breathing unevenly, feeling trapped, frightened and overwhelmed.

The mother breaks down, cries, wants to give up. Contractions are long, hard and close together.

The mother gets a break in contractions, they seem to space out. On the next contraction she is holding her breath and grunting.

The mother is feeling strong urges to push.

The baby is crowning.

The mother is waiting for the placenta to be expelled.

Unit Seven
Self Control

My Thoughts...

Self-Evaluation

Think about your preparations for giving birth.
Do you feel ready? Answer these questions.

	Ready	Almost Ready	Just Beginning
I have identified areas of fear regarding pregnancy, childbirth and becoming a parent.			
I have discussed my fears and concerns with supportive friends and family.			
I have practiced a variety of physical comfort measures for labor.			
I have made a list of the comfort measures most likely to be successful for me during labor.			
I have practiced a variety of positions for labor and childbirth.			
I understand how to use positions and comfort measures to overcome challenges during labor.			
I have discussed the comfort techniques I want to use with my labor support.			
I am getting adequate rest to keep my body as strong as possible.			
I have prepared a bag of labor "tools" including snacks, inspiring quotes, selected music, review sheets of techniques and anything needed for those techniques.			
I have practiced Kegel exercises so I can push effectively.			
I have maintained excellent nutrition to help prevent problems that may hinder a normal birth.			
I have toured my selected birth place and understand the tools available to help me birth normally.			
I have discussed my birth plans with my midwife or doctor.			
I understand what tools my health care provider will use to help labor proceed normally.			
I am ready to speak up for myself, even if it means saying no to something offered by health care providers.			
I agree with my health care providers conditions which will require an induction and methods for induction if necessary.			
I understand the challenges of induction, and am prepared to work through them.			
My support team understands the circumstances in which I will choose to use medications during labor.			
I agree with my health care providers conditions which will require a cesarean surgery.			
My support team understands the circumstances in which I will choose to use cesarean surgery for birth.			

**Unit Seven
Self Control**

My Thoughts...

Is This Labor?

You may not recognize the actual start of your labor. For many women, contractions come and go over a period of days or weeks before actual labor begins. This is normal and expected.

If contractions on and off for days is normal, how do you know when you are actually in real labor? There are a few things you can look for to help you determine what is going on.

First, do not pay attention to the contractions until they demand your attention. Although you may not recognize the moment you move from early labor to active labor, you will recognize the difference between short, mild contractions and the ones that make you stop walking. If you can ignore the contractions, do.

Next, pay attention to how your body responds to physical changes. If your contractions stop when you get up and walk, sit to rest, get a drink or eat something, you are experiencing the normal "before" labor contractions. Try to ignore them and go about your day.

Finally, if you think you are in labor and want to check, pay attention to five or six contractions. See how far apart they are and how long they last. Then, in a few hours pay attention to five or six more. If you are actually moving toward active labor the contractions should be closer together and last longer. You will also notice the intensity of the contractions has increased.

One last important point, your contractions will need to be lasting about sixty seconds in order to make real changes in your cervical dilation. If your contractions are shorter than sixty seconds, try to ignore them.

God's Timing

God's timing is perfect. He knows what you need before you ask. He knows the right time for your baby to be born. He even knows the right amount of labor for your baby.

God provided seven years of great prosperity for the Egyptians which were enough to feed them through the years of famine. It was the job of Joseph to devise a strategy that allowed for the best use of the grain. The food was provided, but with poor stewardship it could have been easily wasted. God did not take the Egyptians out of the famine; he provided for them despite the famine (Genesis 41).

In the same way, God will not take you out of your labor. You will need to experience the time of building pressures and intensity. In the right timing, God will also provide you with tools to help you handle labor. He will give you what you need when you need it, even if it does not seem to be when you thought it should have been available.

Trust God. Let him be in control of the timing of your labor. Let him decide how fast or how slow it should happen. Spend your energy working with the things God has provided for you during labor, recognizing the opportunities he gives you.

Scripture Insight

Read John 14:27, Psalm 29:11 and Psalm 56:3, then answer the following questions.

1. What is peace?

2. What role does peace play in the ability to be self-controlled?

3. Why is self-control important to labor?

4. How do you gain strength?

5. How do you use that strength in difficult times?

To Pray About

Being at peace with God in control.

What have you learned about yourself through labor rehearsals.

Gaining perseverance as you wait for your baby.

Unit Seven
Self Control

My Thoughts...

Control

Ecclesiastes 3:1-5

Isaiah 66:9

Psalm 22:9

Psalm 31:15

Psalm 56:3

Unit Eight
Parenting a Newborn

Overview

As the parent of a newborn, you will be under tremendous pressure from the world to do or provide certain things for your child. You will be met with expectations from those around you, from books and magazines, and from within yourself. Your baby will have needs, and you will do your best to meet those needs. However, you must not allow yourself to become fooled about what those needs really are.

The goal of parenting has never been to provide the perfect meal, best nursery or most educational toys. It is not eternally significant that your baby wait one minute for a diaper change or fifteen minutes. What is eternally significant is that you are an example of the unconditional and sacrificial love of Christ for your child. What is eternally significant is your heart, and your baby's heart. All the details, the little tasks that we feel "must" be done for baby are simply ways to achieve the goal of showing your baby Christ's love.

Discussion Points

- ✓ Let God meet your needs so you will be free to meet your baby's needs.
- ✓ Breast feeding is the healthiest option for most babies. It is also the least expensive and easiest option for most families.
- ✓ Do not compare yourself to someone else. God has given you a unique set of talents and gifts that he expects you to use in life. You will use these gifts in your parenting, so your family may not look like anyone else's.
- ✓ Understanding where your baby is developmentally can help you meet his needs. Babies whose needs are met are best equipped to learn.
- ✓ Be aware of signs of postpartum depression. If your body has any difficulty returning to its normal hormonal balance, your health and your baby's may be at risk because your ability to function well depends on this balance.
- ✓ To have the energy and mental clarity needed for parenting, be sure to continue with good nutrition and exercise.
- ✓ You can use breast feeding time as prayer time, praise and singing time, listening to the Bible on CD, talking to your baby or simply enjoying the break from other duties.

Personal Study

- ❧ Spend an hour "people watching" at a playground or mall. What can you learn from the way parents interact with their young children?
- ❧ Talk to family and friends about feeding newborns. What went well for them and what did not? What can you learn from their experiences?
- ❧ Look through the La Leche League web site or read a book about the basics of breast feeding so you have accurate information to make a decision and are prepared for potential problems if you breast feed.

Scripture Checklist

- ❏ Mark 10:42-45
- ❏ Matthew 20:25-28
- ❏ James 1:5
- ❏ 1 John 4:1
- ❏ 1 Corinthians 4:2
- ❏ Philippians 2:3-8
- ❏ 2 Corinthians 10:12
- ❏ Isaiah 58:11
- ❏
- ❏
- ❏
- ❏

Suggested Readings

Lord of Birth
Becoming a mom

Christian Childbirth Handbook
Newborn Care
Getting to Know Your Newborn
Your new Family

**Unit Eight
Parenting a Newborn
My Thoughts...**

What the Mother May Experience Postpartum

Do you know what to expect after your baby is born? Write an explanation of each topic, and what (if anything) you can do about it.

Shaking

Massage the Fundus

Swelling of the perineum

Soreness

Fatigue

Lochia

Hemorrhoids

Afterbirth Pains

Activity Level

Danger Signs

Heavy bleeding
Fever
Faintness or dizziness
Sharp unexpected pain
"Baby Blues" longer than 2 weeks
Lochia with foul smell
Breast pain
Burning with urination
Inability to urinate
Swollen, red and painful area on leg
Blood clot larger than lemon
Opening of cesarean incision

What Your Baby May Experience

Write in what you need to know about each of these procedures.

APGAR

Vitamin K shot

Eye prophylaxis

PKU test

Vaccinations

Hearing test

Do you know about common newborn characteristics?
What can you expect from your baby in the first few weeks?

Skin

Eyes

Swollen genitals and breasts

Breathing

Bowel movements

Crying

Sleeping

Unit Eight
Parenting a Newborn
My Thoughts...

Unit Eight
Parenting a Newborn
My Thoughts...

Concerns About Your Baby

What might each of these situations mean, and what could you do about it?

No passage of stool within first 24 hours

Sleep periods lasting longer than 6 hours

Hyperirritability (extreme reaction to normal events such as a diaper change)

Jaundice

Poor feeding

Poor color of skin

Labored breathing with grunting

What Your Newborn Needs

Use this space to record a list of the things you think a newborn needs most from parents during the first weeks of life.

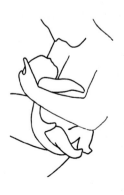

Circumcision

Explore what the Bible says about circumcision.

Genesis 17:10-27

Genesis 21:4

Genesis 34:13-15

Exodus 12:44-48

Leviticus 12:2-4

Deuteronomy 30:6

Joshua 5:2-8

Jeremiah 4:4

Jeremiah 9:25

Acts 10:45

Acts 11:1-18

Acts 15:1-11

Acts 21:17-27

Romans 2:25-27

Romans 4:9-12

1 Corinthians 7:18

Galatians 2:2-4

Galatians 5:2-3

Galatians 6:12-13

Colossians 2:11-12

Colossians 3:11

Find the answers to the following medical questions about circumcision.

1. What is the procedure for circumcision?

2. What is cut off during circumcision?

3. What is the physiological purpose of the part that is cut off?

4. What is done for the pain of circumcision?

5. What care is needed after circumcision?

6. What care is needed for an intact penis?

7. What are the risks of circumcision?

8. What are medical reasons for circumcision?

Unit Eight
Parenting a Newborn

My Thoughts...

**Unit Eight
Parenting a Newborn
My Thoughts...**

The Amazing Newborn

God has created the baby body to respond to life differently than an adult body. These differences provide protection for the baby.

How fast does an adult heart beat?
How fast does a newborn heart beat?
How does this provide protection for a newborn?

How long is an adult sleep cycle?
How long is a newborn sleep cycle?
Why does this provide protection for a newborn?

How often does an adult eat?
How often does a newborn eat?
Why does this provide protection for a newborn?

How does an adult deal with stress or discomfort?
How does a newborn deal with stress or discomfort?
Why does this provide protection for a neworn?

God has created your child complete with personality. Recognizing personality traits in your newborn will give you your first glimpses of who God made him to be. Consider how you will learn the following things about your child's personality.

How easily she adapts to change

How well he handles excessive stimulation

How determined she is

How much help he needs to relax

How willing she is to express herself

How he manages disappointment

How flexible she is with routines

How can you, as a parent, help your child mature into the person God made her to be?

Breast Feeding

Explain what you would tell a new mother about the two most important components of breast feeding:

The Latch

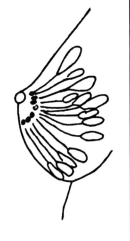

The Position

Breast Feeding Concerns

Find the answers to the following questions.

1. What can you do to help manage engorgement?

2. What helps relieve sore nipples?

3. How can you tell the baby is getting enough to eat?

4. How often should you nurse?

5. How long should you feed on each side?

6. What are common hunger cues in babies?

7. What is a growth spurt?

8. When is it safe to use a supplement?

9. When do babies generally start sleeping through the night?

10. What sources of breast feeding help are in your community?

Unit Eight
Parenting a Newborn

My Thoughts...

Unit Eight
Parenting a Newborn
My Thoughts...

Postpartum Depression

The first 9 months after your baby is born are a time of heightened risk for thyroid dysfunctions. As your body returns to pre-pregnancy hormone levels, you will need to be sure you get plenty of rest and continue your excellent nutrition. If you think you may be experiencing depression, it is important that you seek help immediately. Your health and the health of your baby depend on your body's ability to function well.

Risk Factors

Previous or family history of depression
Major life changes
Lack of social support

Signs to Look for

Crying for no reason
Feelings of apathy or anger about your baby
No longer caring for physical needs of mom or baby
Can not sleep even though you are tired
Loss of appetite
Loss of desire for social contact

Sources of Support

Think about the people in your life who are supporting you now, and those who you expect will support you after your baby is born. To visualize the support, complete this diagram. Make a circle for each person using size to represent how much support you feel they will give you. Then connect the circles to "you."

Support Identification

Now think about all the people you included as sources of support in the previous exercise. What types of support will they be able to give? What types of support will you need? Answer these questions individually, then discuss answers with your loved ones if necessary.

How have you supported yourself during times of stress/change in the past?

What will be your strengths as a parent?

What support do you want from your primary support person?

What support do you want from your family?

What support can you get from the community?

What support will be the most difficult for others to give?

What support will be the most difficult for you to receive?

Unit Eight
Parenting a Newborn
My Thoughts...

Unit Eight
Parenting a Newborn

My Thoughts...

Ministry of Motherhood

Being a parent is as much a ministry as any other work you may choose to do. It requires patience, sacrificial love, perseverance and serving others. However, because the focus of this ministry is our own family, the ministry of motherhood can sometimes feel less important than other works. Have you noticed how we can feel that our best dishes need to be reserved for when guests are visiting? In the same way, some families act as if the way we treat outsiders is more important than the way we treat our spouses and children.

The ministry of motherhood is not about the specific choices you make for your family, but why you make those choices. Are you making decisions to impress others, to make sure your family looks good to outsiders? Or are you making decisions based on meeting the needs of all members of your family, with special consideration for those who need more assistance than others?

There is no blueprint for what a family looks like when you approach motherhood as a ministry. It may mean you work outside the home or inside the home. It may mean you hire a housekeeper, divide chores among family members or do them yourself. It may mean you prepare homemade meals every night or rely on local restaurants.

No two families have the same strengths, challenges and collection of unique members. Avoid the temptation to compare your family to any other family. Instead, compare your family to the ministry God has called you to as a mother.

Parenting

God could have created humankind to live in any manner he felt best suited his creation. He chose families. God chose to have a children cared for by parents for many years before heading out on their own. What value did God see in parenting?

A parent is a godly example to their children. Your unselfish love, practice of forgiveness and willingness to serve demonstrate the life of Christ to your children in a way they could never grasp by merely reading a story. Through your presence, your children will learn how to manage conflict, handle anger and meet the needs of others.

A parent disciples her children. Your loving teaching and correction of your children helps them to learn what it means to be Christ-like. Your attention to your child's growth and maturity help your child discern his gifts and calling from God.

A parent loves his child. The unconditional love of a parent helps children understand the love of God. Acceptance by the parent helps a child to understand they are accepted by God.

Never underestimate the importance of the role you will play in your child's life. Every diaper change you patiently complete, every scraped knee you lovingly mend, every broken heart you tenderly hold teaches your child more than we can imagine.

Scripture Insight

Read Jeremiah 1:5 and Psalm 127:3, then answer the following questions.

1. How does the Bible refer to children?

2. How does your culture view children?

3. When does a child's spiritual life begin?

Read the following laws written to parents. How is each relevant today?

Leviticus 20:1-5

Deuteronomy 12:31

Deuteronomy 13:6-11

Deuteronomy 12:1-15, 17-22; 26-28

Deuteronomy 18:10

Exodus 22:29

Exodus 34:19-20

Deuteronomy 24:16

To Pray About

Your role models for parenting and the choices you will make as a parent.

Your fears about your ability to parent. Pray for faith that God has made you adequate for this task.

Understanding your child's unique personality, with specific gifts, talents and a calling from God.

Unit Eight
Parenting a Newborn

My Thoughts...

New Soul

Jeremiah 1:5

1 Corinthians 12

1 Timothy 4:14

1 Peter 4:10-11

Isaiah 49:15